How to Increase Your Intelligence

by

WIN WENGER

THE BOBBS-MERRILL COMPANY, INC.
Indianapolis/New York

Published by the Bobbs-Merrill Company, Inc.
Indianapolis New York

ISBN 0-672-51786-8

Library of Congress catalog card number 73-1745
Designed by Jacques Chazaud
Manufactured in the United States of America

First printing

Contents

Preface

When the general notion of progress is discussed, we most often refer to the technical innovations man has devised. Our technical abilities allow us to live longer, stay in better health, make toast faster, take pictures on the moon, and, generally, extend our basic capabilities through the use of some technology. But has man really progressed, or has he just benefited from the observation of his own experiences on earth? Has the capability of happiness increased over the last thousand years, and does man have, apart from the tools of his technology, a greater personal potential? The answer is probably negative. And yet the same factors that have given us our great technical advances, namely our thousands of years of living on earth and the attendant accumulation of knowledge, now threaten our existence. If man does not learn to live in peace, he can, by dint of his technology, terminate his existence on earth completely. We have lowered the mortality rates considerably and have found ways of prolonging life through medicine and nutrition, but we are now threatened with problems of overpopulation. And although most countries in the world have made attempts to equalize opportunities among their citizens, we are still hampered by disparities in ability among any given population. The world would undoubtedly be a better place if all the people now alive could understand and utilize the knowledge we presently have. Unfortunately this is not the case, and because it is not, many people are locked into a diminished life style. The reason for this is simple, but painful. Most people cannot use the full potential of intelligence which is available to them. This is what this book is all about: utilizing the full range of human intelligence.

There is a misconception that we are born with a certain intelligence and are trapped forever in the narrow range that is determined to be our "I.Q." The truth of the matter is that unless we are taught to use our brains, unless we understand how our brains work and their relationship to intelligence, we may never even approach truly intelligent functioning. Within all of us is the potential for genius. It is there for us to develop, to explore, and to enjoy. Not only *can* we do this, but in the long run we *must* do this if our society is to dissolve the rapidly piling backlog of problems before they bring us all crashing down.

It is easy to make the subject of intelligence-raising esoteric and complicated, as has been done to so many other fields of human service. When this esotericizing is done, we make the individual overly dependent on the decisions (which often involve factors extraneous to that person's own problem) and expensive services of a few officials and professionals. Our expensive, largely ineffectual and now disintegrating school system is a grim example of what happens when this process is carried through to its logical conclusions.

We badly need such professional services—but to handle special problems, not to conduct people's lives. There are more than enough special problems, and, in any case, only a tiny handful of people are currently trained as professionals in the art and science of intelligence-raising. If we wait for enough professionals to be trained in this field, most of us will have to wait a long time.

A few simple procedures, easily adaptable in every household and institution, could and should have beneficial effects on the intelligence of every child, raising a new generation free of nearly all of the problems, limitations, and failures which so cripple our own times.

At least half of the most convincing information now available on how to raise intelligence can be made easily understandable to the man in the street—enough for him to be able to raise his own intelligence to a major extent, without outside professional help.

If great numbers of people are to enjoy the fruits of this knowledge, there can be no other recourse than this—instructions which can be readily followed by anyone who can read and who, after experiencing successful results, can relate his successes to others.

This book is a formulation of such instructions. In trying to reach many people, we must necessarily present many of the arguments, theories and findings in very broad outline. But even if at some points we have oversimplified (for which we ask the reader's pardon and understanding), we feel that we have included the necessary information every person can use to meaningfully improve his own intelligence. If he wishes to go on once he has done so, he can explore the more formal, esoteric discussions of this subject now available. This book is the beginning, and, perhaps, a means to a richer life.

Introduction Piaget and the Origins of Intelligence

On August 9, 1896, Jean Piaget, the brilliant psychologist and educator, was born in Neuchatel, Switzerland. Educated at the University of Neuchatel, Piaget was to become one of the most influential figures in the field of psychology. His pioneer research on the origins of intelligence improved elementary education in England and changed the direction of psychology throughout the world. This monumental research, however, had humble beginnings. Piaget's first theories, in fact, were based on his own children. He watched them closely as they grew, and even devised little experiments to determine how they understood the world around them and such abstract principles as life and death. Later, as assistant director and then co-director of the Rousseau Institute in Geneva, Piaget expanded his theories as he studied hundreds of other children in informal interviews.

Although the majority of Piaget's research was done in the 1920s and '30s, it did not really begin to affect psychology in America until the 1950s. It was then that his major work on infancy, *The Origins of Intelligence in Children,* was translated into English in this country. Since then, Piaget's theories of intellectual development have revolutionized psychology in America.

According to Piaget, the human mind and nervous system are tools which man uses to adapt to the world around him. This adaptation involves a delicate balance between two processes which Piaget calls "assimilation" and "accommodation." Assimilation occurs when a child relates something new in his environment to his past experiences and existing view of the world. For example, a very young child may point to a cat and exclaim "dog." In this case he is *assimilating* the cat into his concept of "dog"—a furry animal with four legs and a tail. *Accommodation* occurs when new circumstances in a child's environment force him to revise his view of the world to accommodate these new circumstances. If, for example, a child who believes in Santa Claus watches his parents put the gifts under the Christmas tree, he must accommodate himself to this new information and revise his concept of the way Christmas presents are delivered. Intelligence, Piaget feels, is this ability to adapt to the environment.

The adaptive tool, the mind, evolves through a series of stages as it matures from infancy to adulthood. Piaget differentiates four major stages of intelligence: the sensori-motor stage, the preoperational stage, the concrete operational stage, and the stage of formal operations.

The sensori-motor stage lasts from birth to about the age of eighteen months. During this stage, according to Piaget, a child is unable to think of an object unless he is perceiving it at the same time. In other words, if a baby reaches for a toy, and the toy is then covered up, the baby stops reaching for it. As this stage progresses, however, the child's thinking becomes more complex, and he begins to experiment in new situations. He develops a sense of permanence of objects and will begin to look *under* the cover for the toy.

The preoperational stage begins when the child learns to use words to represent objects, and lasts until the child is about seven years old. During this stage the child is extremely egocentric and finds it difficult to take another person's point of view. There is also a tendency to treat objects as symbols of other things. For example, a preoperational-stage child might push a bar of soap around the bathtub as if it were a boat, or climb inside a cardboard carton as if it were a fort. A child in the preoperational stage also tends to judge physical characteristics entirely by appearances. He does not understand that liquids and solids can change shape without changing volume. In Piaget's famous "conservation" experiment, a preoperational-stage child watches a person pour colored water from a short, wide glass into a tall, thin glass. Because the water level is higher in the tall, thin glass, the child believes that it contains more water.

In the concrete operational stage, from ages seven to eleven, a child understands conservation of quantity and relationships between objects. He begins to understand relational terms such as bigger or smaller, lighter or darker. A child in the concrete operational stage has learned many important rules for adapting to the world around him, but he is still unable to cope with abstract reasoning. This ability develops in the final stage of Piaget's model.

The final stage, the stage of formal operations, runs from about age eleven to about age fifteen and is a prelude to adult reasoning. An adolescent in this stage can think in abstract terms and can consider hypothetical situations. He is also able to speculate about the future consequences of his own actions and the actions of others.

According to Piaget, if a child does not have enough experience in one of the stages his development in the following stages might be handicapped. Insufficient experience in one of the stages of development might even prevent a child from reaching an adult level of capabilities. On the other hand, enriching a child's experience in one of the stages should aid his development in the following stages.

On the basis of this theory, Evelyn Sharp has written *Thinking Is Child's Play,* a handbook containing "games" for parents to play with their toddlers. There are games to determine a child's current stage of development and other games, involving such activities as sorting and categorizing, to enrich that stage. Piaget, however, has been alarmed by the way his theories have been used in an effort to speed up development and raise intelligence. He feels that key concepts should not be taught to a child out of sequence. Instead, a child should learn these concepts in their natural order, from his own experience with the world around him. Piaget fears that if a concept is learned out of its natural order, other concepts will be more difficult to learn since they will rest on an artificial basis. If these concepts are learned too early, according to Piaget, the following stages may be damaged. Others believe, however, that a child would not really "learn" these concepts until his insight matured to that point.

To date no experiments have proven that enrichment of a child's developmental stages will speed up the development of his intelligence. Many who have studied Piaget's theories, however, seem to feel that this is the case, but they have not followed up their judgments with I.Q.-correlated tests. Even Piaget himself has done no such studies. His theories, however, are based thoroughly on scientific research and suggest that enrichment of a child's early developmental stages *should* increase his ability to adapt to his environment. This ability to adapt, as we noted earlier, is Piaget's definition of intelligence.

At the Harvard Institute of Cognitive Studies, Jerome Bruner and his associates conducted research that in many ways parallels Piaget's studies. Bruner analyzed the different ways in which individuals learn concepts, beginning in the first, post-natal days of existence. He found that each child develops a characteristic method for learning concepts. This method is largely a function of feedback from what gets results early in the child's interaction with his environment.

Bruner's research involved hundreds of experiments for detecting the nature of thought processes in his test subjects. Through this research Bruner and his associates identified and classified three general types of reasoning, developed sequentially in much the same manner as Piaget's stages. Unlike Piaget's stages, however, all of Bruner's stages remain active and very much a part of adult thinking. The first stages are not superseded by later stages as in Piaget's model.

The earliest level, which corresponds in some degree to the sensori-motor stage and in some degree to the preoperational stage in Piaget's model, Bruner calls "affective (emotional) reasoning." At this level an individual tends to repeat an act because the experiences associated with it feel good, or to avoid an act because the experiences associated with it feel bad. Bruner's second level of reasoning is "functional" or "iconic." To some degree this level corresponds to the stage of concrete operations in Piaget's model. For a child in this stage, a chair is to sit in and a stair is to climb. Engineers and mechanics rely heavily on more sophisticated versions of this mode of thought. Bruner's final, adult level of reasoning, like Piaget's, is "formal," or symbolic.

Bruner suggests that a child's awareness (and, presumably, intelligence) can be increased by teaching him appropriate concepts early in life. He asserts that a child can be taught any idea at any age as long as he is taught in his own vocabulary.

Bruner, like Piaget, sees early enrichment as the key to greater adult awareness. Unlike Piaget, however, he is thinking more in an educator's context than in an environmental one. However, one of Bruner's colleagues at the Harvard Institute of Cognitive Studies, Jerome Kagan, has made some interesting observations about the relationship between perception and the quality of the environment. He sees a need for developmental stimuli to be orderly and distinctive. According to Kagan, if stimuli stand out sharply from a calm background, as in many middle-class homes, perception of the stimuli is more likely. If, however, stimuli are immersed in competing and disagreeably noisy stimuli, which is frequently the case in many slum houses, perception (and development) may be "turned off."

Bruner sees the problem of children's development mainly as a matter of improved schooling. No doubt he would agree with George Crile, Jr.'s, statement: "Given a choice between sending my son to a good college or to a good nursery school, I would choose the nursery school, because that will have a far greater effect on my son's life than any college ever will." Bruner, like Crile, places more emphasis on the lower end of the curriculum.

According to Bruner, a child will develop better awareness if his school curriculum pays great attention to key concepts, teaching these concepts to the child in his own vocabulary and reviewing them in gradually more sophisticated form as that vocabulary increases. But by the time a child enters school his brain and intelligence have almost finished growing, and his intelligence is pretty well set for life. Bruner's studies are insightful, but their practical application is not yet at the level where it would do the most good.

Burton White of Harvard has done many experiments with infants in hospital nurseries. These experiments explored the changes that occur in infant patterns of development when there are experimental changes in the environment. He has found that certain forms of visual enrichment in the nursery accelerated the emergence of some key traits in dozens of infants. It took infants in nonexperimental conditions up to 60 percent longer to exhibit these traits. White's studies, however, cover only a few months of the human life span and do not include any of the traits measured on intelligence tests.

White feels that the primary task of developmental psychology should be to discover the limits of human potential "by continuous matching of optimal environments to emerging abilities." This must be done, according to White, at each stage of life, beginning at birth. "We must ultimately be able to assess the various abilities of a particular child," says White, "and then tailor rearing conditions to suit them."

We now turn to Alfred Kuhn's theories on the subject of developmental psychology. Although his views are one step removed from experimental study, his "armchair" theories are carefully considered hypotheses and predictions.

According to Kuhn, human understanding proceeds by stages much like Piaget's, in which a great deal of experience at any one level is required to develop the "code" for operating at the next level. Kuhn believes that we react to a situation not on the basis of current information alone, but on the basis of the interaction between current information and prior information stored in the brain. Current sensory signals act as cues, triggering related ideas in the brain. Simply understanding that a dolphin is a mammal, for example, gives us a great deal of information both about the dolphin's present biology and habits and about his evolution.

According to Kuhn, we build our conceptual models much as the sciences build theirs. We sort a lot of initial information into concepts or categories; then we build higher-order concepts by working out relationships between those concept-categories. Sometimes what we have been led to expect from our present arrangement of concepts is contradicted by current information, and we resort, from time to time, to revising our categories into new, more useful ones. These categories are the key elements of our "decoding" information. They make it easier for us to handle the billionfold impressions of things which are constantly presented to us by our senses. Incoming information, then, serves only to activate the concepts whose cues most closely correspond to it—concepts which already have most of the details we need worked out. The more appropriate and useful our concepts, the more readily we can understand the world around us.

Enrichment of developmental stages, then, is a key element in the developmental theories of Piaget, Bruner, White, and Kuhn. Piaget's theories suggest that enrichment of the early developmental stages should increase a child's ability to adapt to his environment. Bruner, too, suggests that a child's awareness can be increased by teaching him appropriate concepts early in life. White stresses that we must provide optimal environments at each stage of development, beginning at birth. Finally, Kuhn points out the importance of a great deal of experience at each level of development. The more experience we have with the world around us, the more readily we can understand that world.

This book offers methods of providing the brain, mind, and nervous system with the kind of experience that will allow them to work together more effectively and in better relation to the general environment. In effect, these methods will increase what we know as intelligence.

HOW TO INCREASE YOUR INTELLIGENCE

1 Some Questions at the Start

Are you stuck with the brain you were born with, or can you give yourself a better one?

By using just a few of the techniques described in this book, adults have raised their intelligence ("intelligence" as measured by I.Q. tests, and probably in a broader sense as well) by more than forty points. Persons of average intelligence have managed, after using some of the methods described in this book, to join Mensa.[1]

There are children whose intelligence now tests in the range of genius, some of whom are now in schools for gifted children, who had been so heavily brain damaged, so mentally retarded, that their I.Q. could not be measured. Before some of the methods described in this book were used on them, they were clinically regarded as "human vegetables"; pitied as "mere lumps on the floor." At least one of these children had had half his brain surgically removed. These were exceptional cases, but the particular techniques used on them

1. An international fellowship of highly gifted people from all walks of life. Admission is by intelligence test, in which one must perform better than the 98th percentile to become a member.

have greatly improved the measurable mental and neural abilities of thousands of individuals.

The great leaps in brain-power cited in the above, supposedly exceptional, cases are outrageous in scope and size, but they are fact. Their span dwarfs the difference in intelligence between the "brightest" person you have ever known and the "slowest" person you have ever known. Even a much smaller difference in intelligence than this can mean a world of difference to you. Whatever your goals, most of the methods described in this book must be applied rigorously and simultaneously, jammed together so much that for a while you won't have much time for other things. It will take almost as great an effort to make a small difference in your intelligence as a big difference. You can control the amount of improvement you make in your brain by the length of time you work through a concentrated program of these methods—longer for a big improvement, a shorter period of time for a small one—and you will know fairly quickly, by "feel" and by various self-measurement tests, how much your brain has improved by your efforts.

Why haven't you heard of such happenings before? It seems that these widely scattered methods have seldom been taken into one coherent frame of reference.[2] Scientists researching in widely separated disciplines have made important discoveries but have not successfully coordinated them. Consideration and comparison of these widely scattered discoveries have made evident still other information which few scientists would have suspected. But first let us turn to you, the reader.

When you picked up and opened this book, you had at least three questions in mind:

Can I raise my intelligence?

Why raise my intelligence?

---

2. Except partially, in such books as:
   Hunt, J. McVicker, *Intelligence and Experience* (New York: Ronald Press, 1961).
   Beck, Joan, *How to Raise a Brighter Child* (New York: Trident, 1967).
   Wenger, Win, *On Raising Human Intelligence* (Federalsburg, Maryland: MCM Press, 1971).

How can I raise my intelligence, if indeed it can be raised?

You may have also had a fourth question in mind—what *is* intelligence? You've heard so many different things about what intelligence is that you may not be quite sure—but neither is anyone else sure. Different people mean different things when they say someone is intelligent, bright, smart, or "on the ball." Biologists say that an organism is intelligent if it can take a great deal of its environment into account and use it or adapt to it successfully. Most psychologists and educators use the word *intelligence* to mean whatever it is that intelligence tests or I.Q. tests measure. The designers of those tests pick out various kinds of problem-solving skills which they think best show someone's over-all mental ability (this seems to take in some of what the biologists mean in terms of ability to perceive, to take into account, and to use a wide range of factors), and they design test questions in which one must use those skills to answer correctly.

Despite this wide variety of meanings, nearly everyone who uses the word *intelligence* means some sort of mental ability, alertness, perceptiveness, or awareness involving some function or feature of the brain.

For that matter, measuring the functioning of the brain itself, with electroencephalographs, produces readings which are close to the results given by the best I.Q. tests. The speed with which electrical brain-wave peaks respond to some sudden stimulus such as a flash of light, and the complexity of brain-wave response to that stimulus, tell researchers very nearly what someone's measured I.Q. is.[3]

Our purpose in writing this book is to teach you how to

---

3. As in John Ertl's frequency analyzer, now being popularly marketed. That I.Q. measurement may not be a science is being substantially challenged, however, as in these two papers:

Thomas, Roger K., Jr., *Problems and Procedures in Correlating Electrical Brain Activity With Cognition* (Louisville, Kentucky: Southern Society for Philosophy and Psychology, 1968).

Vogel, W., Broverman, D. M., Klaiber, E. L., Kobayashi, Y., Abrams, G., and Broverman, I. K., *EEG, Androgens and Mental Abilities* (Louisville, Kentucky: Southern Society for Philosophy and Psychology, 1968).

increase intelligence in a basic, biological sense—ability to sense, consider, take into account, and successfully use or adapt to more in your physical, mental, emotional, social, and cultural environments. In the sense we mean it here, to raise someone's intelligence is to let him become a more complete human being; to give him wider-ranging adaptability, heightened awareness and insight, more capacity to respond and to explore. All facets of the human situation involve this basic capacity, not just ability in school or job. Strength, sensitivity, zest, and the power to feel keenly and deeply are as much a part of intelligence, in our meaning of that word, as is the power to reason and symbolize.

To raise your intelligence is to enrich your ability to taste more fully and richly the bittersweet, tragicomic, ugly-beautiful, enthralling, disappointing, exalting, and always fascinating experience of being human.

At first glance this *seems* to be a long way from what most readers likely had in mind when they picked up this book: a wish to succeed better at job or school. If you want to raise your intelligence to do better in school, keep in mind that, as schools now teach, intelligence and success in school have little in common. As-yet unquantified experience with large numbers of people who have had to work at increasing their mental abilities[4] does suggest that by building up your intelligence, you *probably* will do at least somewhat better in school. If you are trying to be more successful in your occupation, you may be better helped by most of this book, because intelligence and career success do have something in common. Still, many other factors enter into success, and as you become more intelligent, you will become interested in other things besides career success; this may change some of your goals. This book will help you to some extent, whatever your purpose; it will

4. Together with other groups using their methods, The Institutes for the Achievement of Human Potential, 8801 Stenton Avenue, Philadelphia, Penna. 19118, have gathered experience with more than twelve thousand brain-damaged and/or mentally retarded patients, curing a substantial majority of them. Most of these were children who were later placed in school.

help you *most* if your goal is, straightforwardly, that of becoming a more intelligent human being.

At first glance, this is also a long way from simply raising intelligence as measured on I.Q. tests. The broader, more basic, biological meaning of *intelligence* is hard to measure. There *are* ways to raise your scoring on I.Q. tests without doing much to your fundamental intelligence—these ways don't interest us very much, although we will have a little to say about them later. *If* you can raise your intelligence to any real extent, you will most likely raise your I.Q. scores considerably, and this will mean a lot more than would your raising I.Q. scores without boosting real intelligence.

This book will also be a great help to you if your interest is that of raising the intelligence of your child (which is somewhat easier than raising the already-established intelligence of an adult). Further, we will draw your attention to other books which will also help you in boosting your child's capabilities.

Practically no one in the sciences uses the word *intelligence* to mean "broad acquaintance with a lot of facts," and you will find that most scientists' definitions of *intelligence* are very far from this common, man-in-the-street use of the word. You may develop or improve such an information background, both as a direct result of improving your basic ability to acquire and use information and as a byproduct of several of the intelligence-raising methods suggested in this book. Being well informed may be a *result* of intelligence; it is not what scientists mean by *intelligence* as such, and most modern intelligence tests have been redesigned to better measure intelligence as basic ability *separate from* one's particular cultural background.

Several things have until recently discouraged most scientists from examining the question of whether human intelligence can be raised. One is the opinion that intelligence is inborn, bred into the genes—that you are stuck with the brain you were born with and there's precious little you can do about it. If people believe that intelligence is inborn, they are forced to respond to the question in one of several ways:

Steer clear of questions of intelligence or else you must be an elitist or, when dealing with I.Q. differences between races, a bigot. If I.Q.s can't be meaningfully changed, then to dwell on the subject of intelligence would be to dwell on something which makes one race permanently superior or inferior to another—or so the thinking goes. Actually, differences in *average* racial I.Q. mean nothing with respect to any particular individual's intelligence; every human group has both geniuses and idiots, and a lot of people scattered between those extremes. So long as intelligence is thought to be inborn and unchangeable, however, the *feeling* of a racial slur is there every time the subject of intelligence comes up. If, though, intelligence is changeable, and markedly affected by things other than heredity, the question of race is replaced by that of living conditions, and that matter has a wholly different feeling to it. And by living conditions I mean more than simple environment. Other responses likely if people feel that intelligence is inborn and unchangeable—

If you are of high intelligence, do not admit it and don't even use it much, or you will be considered a snob harping on something that is unfair to other people and which they can't do anything about.

If you are not of high intelligence, then you have an excuse for not getting very far in life.

Or, if you are not of high intelligence, intelligence can't be anything that matters very much; people would be better off without it.

Talking about inborn and unchangeable advantages or disadvantages is useless—it can only spoil the advantaged and discourage the disadvantaged. If intelligence is inborn and unchangeable, it's a pointless subject to dwell on.

All these and other harmful attitudes about the subject, which have kept many scientists from examining the question of whether human intelligence can and should be improved, have a bearing only so long as people believe that intelligence is both inherent and unchangeable. If more people realized how readily human intelligence can be improved, intelligence-raising would be widely seen as the finest, noblest, and most useful thing anyone could do. Your experience can help bring about this change in attitude. When, through your example, people discover that intelligence can be earned, some will realize, as others have, that to develop fuller human capabilities in oneself and in others is one of the very highest and finest of callings.

2
Yes: You Can Raise Your Intelligence

The only apparent limit on how successfully you can raise your own intelligence, given presently available techniques, is your will to do so.

You can improve your own brain as far as you want to. But whatever the techniques used, it takes a lot of effort and hard work.

Consider the seat of human intelligence—the human brain. Every mode of behavior, response, ability, whatever it is that any of us call intelligence, is based on the physical state of the brain and its physical processes.

The brain and its workings are physical—as physical as your heart or liver, and so can be changed by physical processes. For example, you can improve the brain's working condition by improving the brain's circulatory lifeline.

In any encyclopedia or physiology text you will find described a pair of arteries—the carotids—which convey life-giving oxygenated blood and nutrition to the brain (the jugular veins carry "soiled" blood from the brain back to the heart for recirculation). Without the carotids, no blood, oxygen, or food could reach the brain.

Klosovskii[1] and other noted brain scientists note that only those brain cells which are near to ample capillary blood supply are developed. Away from such source of supply, brain cells remain undeveloped and useless. Albert Einstein's genius turned out to result largely from extra circulatory functioning in his brain, not from extra brain matter. His brain, better nourished, worked better. You can give yourself similarly enhanced circulation in your brain to give it extra oxygen and nutrition to run on. In short, you can much improve the physical state of your entire brain. You can do this because of one special feature of those carotid arteries which supply the brain—the valves of those arteries, located in the back of the neck.

These carotid valves open wider to let more blood flow past whenever there is a momentary increase in the carbon dioxide content of the bloodstream. If this momentary CO_2 increase happens very frequently, it "trains" these valves to open wider permanently and let more through to the brain, building up the brain's circulatory system and thus the physical well-being of your entire brain.[2] Combine this "CO_2 training" of the carotid valves with specific nutritional elements associated with development of the capillaries, with expansion of flow capacity of capillaries, veins, and arteries, with reduction of oxygen need, as cited in our chapter on nutrition, and with the other procedures, described further on in this book, which will help newly supplied brain cells to develop—and you will indeed improve the physical condition and physical workings of your brain. You will have given yourself a better

---

1. Klosovskii, B. N., *The Development of the Brain, and its Disturbance by Harmful Factors* (Elmsford, New York: Pergamon, 1963).

2. CO_2-training the carotid valves has become perhaps the most important element in the program used by Philadelphia's Institutes for the Achievement of Human Potential to cure brain damage, mental retardation, and reading disabilities, and to otherwise raise the intelligence and improve the brain functioning of thousands of patients.

basis for all your thinking, seeing, hearing, feeling, emotions, sense of beauty, awareness, comprehension, memory, aspiration—for your brain is what perceives, and holds, all your experiences—is the organ which maintains and operates your entire physical body as well, incidentally—and is the seat of all that anyone means when he refers to "intelligence."

How can you CO_2-train your carotid valves to let more through to your brain? Of many possible ways, the one liked best by the researchers who developed this approach[3] is called masking. Rebreathe your own breath from a bag for a half minute, every half hour. A medium-sized grocery bag will do. Though probably no one has ever suffocated or could possibly suffocate in a paper grocery bag, in view of the trouble young children had with plastic bags a few years back, take these precautions: insert a soda straw or other small tube through a hole in the bag, and/or have someone else around, and/or don't run the rebreathing sessions for longer than a half minute at a time.

Such precautions notwithstanding, masking is an easy method, costs nothing (by contrast, CO_2 treatments at hospitals using twenty-thousand-dollar machines cost around a hundred dollars per session), but presents some social difficulty. You can hardly whip out a paper bag at work or school every half hour and say, "Excuse me a minute, I've got to mask," without drawing some very odd reactions from your co-workers or schoolmates.

This social difficulty is one reason why you should squeeze most of your brain-boosting into a several-week vacation session rather than spreading it out through the year. Even if you could plead sinus or stomach disorders as an excuse to disappear to the bathroom every half hour, there are other, more important reasons (which we will discuss later) for jamming your brain-boosting into a very concentrated several weeks. Masking *should* be done every half hour during work-

3. Philadelphia's Institutes for the Achievement of Human Potential.

ing or school hours over such a concentrated period rather than more frequently or stretched out over longer intervals. In practice, this half-hour interval appears to have given the best results. Here, as in so many other aspects of intelligence-raising in adults, halfway measures don't give half the results; they give next to no results at all. The concentration of half-hour intervals is important.

Another way to CO_2-train your carotid valves to let more through to your brain is hold-your-breath-type underwater swimming. Forcing yourself many times in each daily swim session to stay under water longer and longer before coming up to breathe would, in a month or so of such daily sessions, help make up in intensity for the lack of frequency (frequency as compared with the masking every half hour during waking hours). Individuals have, without knowing it at the time, greatly enhanced their mental abilities by such underwater sport.

Of course you could also expel your breath and hold it out for a half minute every half hour, and do this even during everyday activities and especially during exercise. But without something as attention-holding as coming up from under water, or as concrete as a paper bag, such simple expelled-breath-holding seems to be psychologically much more difficult to keep up for the days and weeks necessary to produce the desired effect.

Jogging or other respiration-stimulating exercise each day also has some effect on the carotid valves and thus on the brain. Like the underwater swimming, jogging benefits your entire physical body, including your brain. But jogging's direct effects on the physical well-being of the brain have not been shown to be as notable as the direct effects on the brain of simple masking.

Mysterious as many features of the human brain still are to us, here at least there is no mystery. Using CO_2 enrichment to expand your brain's circulatory system is a perfectly straightforward physical way to improve the physical bases of your intelligence.

Because your brain is a physical organ in your body, affected by the physical conditions in which it works, you can make physical improvements in your brain by such means. Like any other part of your physical body, its well-being and functioning depend on how much life-giving oxygen and nutrition its cells get, and masking, underwater swimming, jogging, and even other forms of exercise directly affect this. In chapter 4 we will have more to say about nutrition and ways to improve the physical condition of your whole brain by means other than those that depend on retraining your carotid valves.

Like so many of the techniques to be cited in this book, the technique we call masking is quite easy—just rebreathing your own breath in a paper bag, now and then. What's hard about it is continuing to do it, over and over, every half hour, for several weeks, and finding time to do it without having problems with curious co-workers or friends. It takes more determination to carry through than many people—perhaps most people—have, even though the method itself is so easy. Or perhaps even *because* the method is so easy?

But by understanding the workings of those CO_2-sensitive carotid valves in the back of your neck you can actually see *why* simple masking improves your brain and intelligence.

This makes somewhat academic much of the argument as to *whether* you can raise your intelligence. However, because so many people think you cannot, including most experts who should know better, we will deal with at least some of the argument.

The main belief appears to be that intelligence is inborn and hereditary. That there is a hereditary component to intelligence we certainly agree: one can even breed "bright" and "dull" strains of the same stock of animals, and human intelligence varies over a wider range than that of other animals. But it's doubtful that anyone would hold the opinion that if an infant with the brain potential of an Albert Einstein had been chained to a bedpost in the attic for all of his growing-up years, he would have become an intelligent adult. That beautifully potentialed Einstein would have been a drooling idiot. So even the most adamant believers in the hereditarist theory of intelligence agree that environment has at least something to do with the way intelligence is formed.[4]

Especially after the orphanage studies of Spitz,[5] Dennis,[6] Hunt,[7] and others, showing the pitiful retardation which results in human children who lack environmental stimulus; the hospital nursery studies of Burton White,[8,9] which showed

---

4. Many supporters of the theory that intelligence is mainly hereditary cite various I.Q. studies of identical twins who were separated at birth and raised in different families. The most that such twins differed usually ran about 15–20 points I.Q. Hereditarists overlook these two points in their own argument, however:

   (1) 15–20 points I.Q. is nevertheless a very large difference in someone's life, consciousness, career possibilities, and many other things. To go up 15–20 points on the I.Q. scale, other things being equal, is probably to double or treble the actual quantity of intelligence and to increase by several orders of magnitude the scope of things which one can do or be aware of.

   (2) All the studies were taken with the twins still in the same culture. No matter how big the differences within our culture, the ways we are all alike are far more important when contrasted to other cultures. Our culture is far too uniform to allow very great differences in I.Q. to show up via random-factor studies of identical twins. I.Q. differences many times greater than this 15–20 points can be readily produced by specific changes in the environment.

5. Spitz, René A., "Hospitalism: An Inquiry into the Genesis of Psychiatric Conditions in Early Childhood," Eissler, R. S., Freud, A., Hartman, H., and Kris, E. (eds.), *The Psychoanalytic Study of the Child,* Vol. I (New York: International University Press, 1945).

6. Dennis, W., "Causes of Retardation Among Institutional Children: Iran," *Journal of Genetic Psychology,* XCVI, 1960.

7. Hunt, J. McVicker and Archer, Forough Minou, "An Experimental Study of Psychological Development Before and After Auditory and Visual Enrichments of Orphanage Experience in Young Infants (draft of plan for the program)." Private monograph.

8. White, Burton L., "An Experimental Approach to the Effects of Experience on Early Human Behavior," Hill, J. P. (ed.), *Min-*

adequately stimulated human infants developing at twice the rate of other infants who did not receive stimulation; and the seemingly endless succession of laboratory studies by David Krech and his colleagues varying the intelligence of laboratory animals across the entire range of intelligence as measured within the species involved—especially after these and hundreds of other well-documented scientific studies on these points over the past three and a half decades, even the most ardent supporter of the hereditarist theory of intelligence admits that intelligence emerges as a product of the interplay of hereditary nature with environment.

Even admitting that intelligence emerges as a product of the interplay of hereditary nature with environment, most opinion still holds that genetic heredity decides 80 to 90 percent of what your I.Q. is; that the environment around you accounts for only 10 percent, perhaps 20 percent at best.

That this consensus has not been very well thought out can be shown by the simple question: What percent of the outcome of play at second base in the game of baseball is due to the thrown ball? What percent of the outcome is due to the fielder? The base runner? Like the majority opinion just cited, such questions are meaningless.

To ask what portion of the outcome is due to one of those factors at second base means nothing—it is the *interplay* of those factors which matters, and the outcome of that interplay, like that of the interplay between heredity and environmental factors which form intelligence, can vary all over the ballpark. The runner can be safe, or out, or retreat successfully to first base, or be caught in a run-down, or advance still farther on an error, or have his teammate make it across home plate

---

nesota Symposium On Child Psychology (Minneapolis: University of Minnesota Press, 1967).

9. White, Burton L. and Held, H., "Plasticity of Sensorimotor Development in the Human Infant," Rosenblith, J. F. and Allinsmith, W. (eds.), *The Causes of Behavior: Readings In Child Development and Educational Psychology* (Boston: Allyn and Bacon, 1966).

during the action at second base—all these widely different outcomes, and more, with the same ingredients. It all depends on how those ingredients interplay, interact, relate to one another. The same ingredients—but such differing results depending on who, or what, gets to second base first!

The same is true with human intelligence. As we have seen, even the most ardent supporters of the theory that heredity is the main basis of intelligence admit that this intelligence is a product of the interplay of an individual's genetic, hereditary nature with his surroundings. As with the play at second base, therefore, and as in any case where you have the product of interplay, the outcome can vary greatly even with the same ingredients. The interplay of the same factors can produce an I.Q. of 50 or an I.Q. of 150—the difference between low-grade moron and near-genius.

That this simple fact could have eluded so many learned authorities for so long is astounding, but there it is.

Clearly, environment is not everything: there must be something there for it to work on. Heredity can and does make key differences. But for intelligence to grow, it must be fed: it must feed on a psychologically nourishing environment. One may use environment to raise or lower intelligence to an enormous extent few people have as yet begun to realize.

Anyone who still thinks of intelligence as basically a fixed, hereditary quantity has some interesting problems to face. For example, compared to I.Q. scores taken under usual test conditions, what would be the result of an I.Q. test taken by the same person immediately after a thunderingly successful Thanksgiving dinner? Or after he put his brain temporarily into "high gear" with extra dosages of choline and vitamin B-12? Which is his "true" I.Q.?

If the quantity which traditional psychologists call intelligence does in fact show up in I.Q. scores, should we then assume that it does *not* show up in that post-turkey score? If we must say that such easily brought about differences in the test subject's physical condition account for those differences in his I.Q. test scores, should we then turn around and say that other, also easily brought about differences in the physical conditions of several individuals have nothing to do with the measured I.Q. differences between those individuals?

To say that such easily brought about differences in physical condition have nothing to do with intelligence is to throw away not only the standard definition of intelligence "as that which is measured on I.Q. tests," but all accepted scientific definitions of intelligence, in favor of some mystic, unknown quality which has no basis of measurement.

Whoever tries to say that changing physical conditions will not change intelligence must therefore assume the burden of responsibility for redefining intelligence in scientifically measurable terms, if his opinion that intelligence is a fixed, unchangeable, mainly heredity-based quantity is to hold any validity at all.

On much the same grounds we may ask: What is the I.Q. of someone who is unconscious, or in a coma, or conscious but dazed, or fully awake but with faculties temporarily deranged by a stroke, a head blow, chemicals, or a strong impulse of emotion . . . or who is intoxicated, or who is suffering a high fever . . . or who is dead? What can we say of the unchangeable intelligence of any one person who, at one time or another, undergoes all these conditions?

Supposing the traditional expert, still arguing for an hereditarist view, backtracks and says, "Agreed that very large differences in the physical condition of someone may have something to do with the way his I.Q. is expressed. But most people, at most times, are in reasonably good physical condition, and so we can assume, for the most part, that intelligence is what would be expressed by a person's brain and nervous system if he were at his best."

Are most people, here in flabby America, in reasonably good physical condition most of the time? Your answer probably is *No!*

Do we even know what someone's top physical condition would be? If somehow we did, could we even know to what extent this difference from that top condition would affect his I.Q. scores?

No one has even the slightest notion of what would be expressed by the brain and nervous system of someone at his best—no one in our experience, or even in history, has come close to it.

That "best" is so far beyond what could be measured by our present I.Q. tests as to make them quite meaningless, and with them the traditional expert's own arguments based on them. For example:

The average human has ten to twenty billion brain cells. Only about 5 percent of these brain cells are at all developed, matured beyond the preinfantile, undeveloped, nonfunctioning condition at which they began.[10,11,12] Of those paltry few cells which are developed to any extent, most have only a few hundred, or even a few dozen, circuit connections with other cells. Yet some of these developed brain cells have been found to have up to twenty *thousand* connections,[13] and no doubt brain cells could develop several times this number of such links.

It is not enough to say that the human brain is only five to ten percent developed, the portion of its available cells which have come into any use at all. When one takes into account the number of connections between those few developed cells, the difference between actual and potential development becomes immense.

One can no longer say that the human brain is only five percent developed. He can no longer say that the human brain

---

10. Young, J. Z., *A Model of the Brain* (London: Oxford University Press, 1964).

11. Eccles, J. C., "Possible Ways in Which Synaptic Mechanisms Participate in Learning, Remembering, and Forgetting," *The Anatomy of Memory: Proceedings of the First Annual Conference on Learning, Remembering, and Forgetting* (Palo Alto, California: Science and Behavior Books, 1965).

12. Klosovskii, B. N., *The Development of the Brain, and Its Disturbance by Harmful Factors* (Elmsford, New York: Pergamon, 1963).

13. Young, *op. cit.*

is one percent developed. He cannot even say that the human brain is one thousandth, or even one millionth, of one percent developed!

And we now know of many ways to "turn on" brain cells, develop them, extend their connections, their usability. If, using these, you even made yourself into a genius, you would only be raising the fulfillment of your potential from perhaps one trillionth to one and a third trillionth.

Our real development compared to our potential is like a grain of sand compared to a beach: in seeking a second grain of sand to go with the first, does it really matter that much whether that beach of heredity is five miles long and a hundred yards wide, or three miles long and fifty yards wide?

While straining at gnats (or, if you prefer, at grains of sand), our traditional experts have, I fear, swallowed quite a few camels. Though we have argued the matter more extensively elsewhere,[14] on just these few grounds cited above there can remain very little doubt that the popular notion that intelligence is a fixed, hereditary, unchangeable quantity is in serious error. It is evident that intelligence can in fact be raised or lowered, *has in fact been* raised and lowered by various factors in your environment, and, as we shall see in the next chapter, *should* be raised.

On that beach of potential, there are plenty of grains of sand to go after.

---

14. Wenger, Win, *On Raising Human Intelligence,* Chapter 2 (Federalsburg, Maryland: MCM Press, 1971).

3
Why Should You Improve Your Brain?

The next time you get a chance to gaze at a glorious sunset, its patterns and gradations of almost every beautiful color known to man encompassing the entire horizon and giving such life to the immense sky over you that your throat aches . . . next time you gaze at a sunset like that, imagine yourself color-blind and viewing the same scene.

"Very interesting," the color-blind person would say to his companion, shrug, and turn back inside. The oceanic beauties of that sky hold very little of interest for his eyes, even though he's looking at the same scene you are.

Walking down a street the next day, you muse on the sad plight of your friend. "How drab it must be to live in a world in which you cannot see color!" you think as you walk past an art gallery filled with Rubens and Michelangelo and Picasso and Dali, trudge unnoticing by habit past a library filled with texts on astronomy and physics and economics, with volumes of Shakespeare and Whitehead and Roethke, with records and tapes of Bach and Hindemith, Schubert and Stravinsky.

"Think of looking at a sunset like that," you muse, "and not seeing the color. Of not even being interested." Passing the group of children at play on the corner, you fail to note the highly visible signs of nutritional deficiency in one and, in another, a neurological deficiency which if not soon corrected will place its victim beyond the pale of mainstream humanity. Arriving at work or school, you miss the increasing signs of stress in one of your co-workers or fellow students which evidences something which, because you didn't know, will soon cost you his friendship. "Actually seeing the same thing I was looking at," you wonder, "but not really seeing it at all. Amazing!"

The vast majority not only of the great discoveries and great inventions, but of the great arts, the recorded impressions of beauty and human feeling and experience—two thirds or more of all of these vital gardens of culture and civilization were contributed by a mere handful of gifted individuals.[1]

By far the greater part of such human experience, perception, feeling, and awareness as has been recorded was recorded by the highly intelligent—and a lot of it *for* the highly intelligent. True, the greatest things that mankind's greatest geniuses had to say are great *because* they say something meaningful to nearly all of us. Yet there is so much *more* in what they said than what most of us read!

After all, in the greatest sunsets even the color-blind can see that there's an interesting pattern of light in the sky. Maybe your color-blind friend will even enjoy, after a fashion, that (to him, gray) pattern of light in the sky.

Becoming more intelligent enables you to contact more of mankind. To share more of the human experience. To touch those roots of what mankind's finest members feel are the essentials of the experience of being human.

Try an experiment. Pick a painting or a piece of classical music, one you haven't paid much attention to before but which you like. Study it closely; see how much you can enjoy it. Then read some articles or a book on that piece of art and its creator, some well-informed criticism and description.

1. Cox, Catherine M., "The Early Mental Traits of Three Hundred Geniuses," *Genetic Studies of Genius,* Vol. II (Stanford: Stanford University Press, 1926).

Finally, go back to that painting or piece of music. What's your experience of that piece of work like now?

You could get the same effect from looking around your by now all-too-familiar neighborhood if you could find someone intelligent enough or poetic enough to analyze and/or describe it well for you.

What story, essay, poem, or book that you read five or even ten years ago, of those you enjoyed, do you think had the most to say to you? Reread it now. What more is it saying to you now?

If you saw either of the movies *Blowup* or *2001,* see the film again when it comes around on reruns. What do you see this time?

If "mere" experience can do these things for you, what can higher intelligence do?

Today there are ways to feed electrical stimuli directly to "pleasure centers" in the brain. To do so creates intense feelings of pleasure which can be sustained indefinitely, and without any harm whatever. You've heard people say that all they wanted in life was enough pleasure to be happy with. Well, they are wrong even about themselves—that is *not* all they want, and the next paragraph will probably prove it to you:

Given the choice between continuing to experience life as you are doing, and retiring to some dark closet without respite for the rest of your life as the condition for perpetual and absolutely harmless deep pleasure, even ecstasy, by permanent stimulation of your pleasure center—given that choice, you know, we all know, which you will choose. Even those of your friends who say that all they want of life is some pleasure will make the same choice that you did.

Why?

Why would you spurn that Eden of an offer—of spending the rest of your life in a padded closet with a "whoopee cap"?

Because *all* of us basically want to perceive, to know, to be aware, to experience. We want to live, not just be pleased. And living is experiencing. The more completely we experience, the fuller our lives become. Society may have punished most of us out of our curiosity, our drive to know things, our unashamed appreciation of beauty, our readiness to come up with new ideas and new ways—but in almost none of us has society totally extinguished this basic wish and need found in all of us, the drive to be *sentient*.[2]

Sensory-deprivation experiments tell us that man and all higher mammals desperately need some experiencing at all times—without it, they will start hallucinating experiences. Then they will go insane. Then, sometime later, they will die.

The drive to be sentient is that basic to us. Superficially, society may have conditioned us to think that all we really want is money, or sex, or pleasure, or peace. But society cannot really extinguish that basic drive to be sentient, of which power, sex, pleasure, etc., are but such feeble expressions, without extinguishing *us* as well.

Realizing this basic drive, you can now begin to go after what you really want. And in addition, becoming more sentient, more intelligent, can serve as a tool for you to attain more readily whichever of those more superficial but desirable things you also want—including that greater success at school or on the job, if that is your goal.

But, you might say, being deprived of anything makes that thing more important. Being deprived of air, for example, will quickly make your need for air much more important than all your other needs put together. I may have *a* drive to be sentient, as you say, but do I have a basic drive to be *more* sentient? Why wouldn't I want to settle for having average or normal intelligence? Some answers to this point:

1) You are correct about unmet needs taking on greater importance. This is why it is necessary to develop the *whole* person, in this or any other program. Just the narrow abilities to reason logically and to symbolize, or to have a larger vocabulary—bases of some I.Q.-raising schemes—just aren't

2. Students of many disciplines might find it useful to talk about "sentiles"—units of sentience—in a quantitative manner even when we have no real measure of that quantity, just as students of economics, political science, and strategy theory found it quintessentially useful to talk about units of pleasure—"utiles"—at a time when no way existed to measure that quantity.

satisfactory. The amputated hand or foot still itches, still hurts, years after. So also the amputated parts of your psyche itch you, bother you. Those parts of you which *weren't* developed will keep making you uncomfortable from time to time.

2) When you were a child you certainly evidenced the drive to be *more* sentient, until it was conditioned out of you so thoroughly that you don't even recognize that unsatisfied drive as the source of occasional discomfort and the secret conviction that something is missing.

3) If nearly everyone, including you, were color-blind, but a few people weren't and could see the colors and beauties of the sunset, sunrise, fresh green countryside, fabrics, and you knew of a way to begin to perceive colors, wouldn't you want to use that way? . . . Or, maybe you wouldn't. If, somehow, you *don't* have that drive, then there are still many practical reasons why you should want to raise your intelligence—but it would certainly be a pity.

4) If you want "normal" intelligence, then you certainly *don't* want "average" intelligence. "Normal" is *not* "average." "Normal" means whole, intact, healthy; "average" reflects all the ills and sick conditions and scars that most people bear. Let us illustrate the difference this way:

Picture a strange, exotic island where the practice is to cut off every child's right arm at birth. When all those children reach adulthood, they will be average in relation to that island's inhabitants in physical configuration—but will they be normal? The unhappy fact is that many ordinary practices of our culture are the equivalent of cutting off every baby's right arm.

We are nearly all significantly brain damaged. Standard American obstetric practices are associated with much of that damage—anesthesia or analgesia to the mother in labor, placing her horizontally instead of vertically for delivery of her child, and numerous other practices cited elsewhere.[3,4,5] Even

3. Dick-Read, Grantly, *Childbirth Without Fear* (New York: Harper and Row, 1944).

in the better metropolitan hospitals, studies show that we are so badly damaged at birth that the brains of 80 percent of us bleed for hours afterward.[6]

Developmentally we are damaged as well. Anything interfering much with our creeping and crawling around as infants, such as a playpen or a fastidious mother or nurse who would have been shocked at the idea of letting Baby down on the dirty old floor, damages us directly. This lack of creeping and crawling is directly and closely associated with visual, reading, and writing problems, and most of us who aren't handicapped greatly by it are usually handicapped at least a little, but without knowing it. Other household practices and circumstances also hinder our development. Indeed, the problem is so general and so vast that if you do want a normal intelligence, as contrasted to an average intelligence, you want an intelligence far higher than even the procedures in this book can give you. But you may have some reason for wanting only an average intelligence, sick and maimed as such an intelligence is, because:

Being highly intelligent does carry with it some problems. It is not entirely a bed of roses; there are thorns.

Being exceptionally intelligent is like being the only one of the passengers on the ship of life to notice that the ship is veering uncontrolled into a field of icebergs—and being unable to get anyone else to see or notice it. It's like noticing a cliff face sparkling with diamonds—and being unable for

---

4. Calkins, Leroy A., *Normal Labor* (Springfield, Illinois: Charles C Thomas, 1955).

5. Guttmacher, Alan F., *Pregnancy and Birth* (New York: Viking, 1956). Further criticisms of standard obstetric practice are referred to in chapter 3 of Wenger, Win, *On Raising Human Intelligence* (Federalsburg, Maryland: MCM Press, 1971).

6. The writer is apprised, by Dr. Glenn Doman of Philadelphia's Institutes for the Achievement of Human Potential, of a study conducted in a major hospital there by Dr. Eugene Spitz revealing blood in 800 of the spinal taps he conducted on 1,000 consecutive newborn infants.

a long, exasperating while to persuade anyone that the boat should pull over and investigate it. Being very intelligent brings some loneliness—none of your fellows share certain of your interests and perceptions, and all are unaware that much of your world even exists. Even if you make your fellows look closely at what you have discovered to be a pearl of inestimable value, all they see is a dull blob . . . *but:*

Even these aspects of high intelligence have their rewards. You, at least, do get to gaze upon that pearl. Your world is open, interesting, adventurous, fascinating, intricate, at some points incredibly beautiful. You may or may not persuade that boat to put over for the diamond-studded cliff, but if you can swallow your frustration and remember its location, you can come back later and reap it. If you can't persuade anyone to notice the ship of life careening toward icebergs, you can ensconce your loved ones and yourself in a life raft and have a good chance of coming through the worst. And maybe, just maybe, you can find someone else highly intelligent with whom to share your special world.

There are many immediately practical reasons why you should seek to improve your brain, in addition to the foregoing discussion of why you really want to do so.

The person of truly 140 I.Q. can be a ditchdigger, a plumber, a poet, a lawyer, a physician—by choice. The person of truly 70 I.Q. can be a ditchdigger—no choice. In an age of cybernetics, when machines are increasingly able to handle all repetitive work, ditchdiggers have less and less reason to stay alive, and the current political swing in our country indicates that welfare recipients, the former ditchdiggers, will have fewer and fewer means of subsistence.

Very simply, the range of careers open to a person of high intelligence tends to be very wide, although of course other variables enter in, such as work attitude, level of schooling, social advantages, etc. Similarly, in most careers the level of achieved position in later years also correlates highly with intelligence—as does the length of time one has to enjoy and pursue a career in the first place, since intelligence correlates so highly with one's physical condition and lifespan. Many studies indicate that how long you live, as well as how well you live, relates closely to how intelligent you are.

Severely brain-damaged patients brought by the thousands to Philadelphia's Institutes for the Achievement of Human Potential had all the health problems and poor life-length prospects of mental retardates everywhere. As this brain damage and retardation was cured and these patients' intelligence rose, their health improved tremendously and their physical condition was strikingly transformed.[7]

This is not very surprising: the brain controls every aspect of the body. Improve much in the way one part of the brain functions, and you make some improvement in all of the brain's functioning.[8] The better the brain functions, the better off is the body it maintains—no wonder that more than forty years of careful research at Stanford University show that more often than not, it is the intellectually gifted person who is also physically stronger, healthier, nimbler, and more attractive.[9]

All the continuing, persisting problems you face, or that society faces, by definition remain problems because not enough intelligence has been marshaled to solve them. Raising your own intelligence may not solve all your problems, but it should increase your ability to do so.

Greater success obtainable in career, improved schoolwork, longer, healthier life, greater ease in solving your present problems—a host of solidly practical reasons exist for you to raise your intelligence.

There is yet one more reason why you should raise your

---

7. On the records of, at last count, 13,000 brain-damaged patients treated via the Institutes for the Achievement of Human Potential in Philadelphia, or via affiliated institutes elsewhere using much the same procedures.

8. LeWinn, Edward B., *Human Neurological Organization* (Springfield, Illinois: Charles C Thomas, 1969).

9. Terman, Lewis M., *Genetic Studies of Genius* (Stanford: Stanford University Press, volumes continuing since 1926).

intelligence: others need you. Our society needs you as a more intelligent person. Our intelligence has not been great enough to solve the problems which have disrupted our society and environment and threatened an actual end to life itself on Earth, by many different routes of disaster. Our intelligence *must* be raised soon. There is no choice.

Whether you yourself, as a more intelligent person, play any active role in solving these larger problems, your better brain will act as a leaven on those around you, easing the severe handicap which an unintelligent public, by its very being, places on those of our public-policy makers who seek intelligent solutions to our problems. Many times that handicap has proven very damaging. As your brain's improved abilities influence people around you, your effect on such problems, even without your attention on them, will be much greater than the proportion of "one man—one vote."

Whether you care about such larger matters, you still have all those practical, personal reasons to raise your intelligence. And you have powerful basic reasons for wanting to grow back some of that seeing-feeling-hearing-thinking-acting part of yourself that was amputated from you long ago.

One last thing not yet mentioned: when one is in top form and physically strong, he rejoices in the use of his strength. It feels very good to exercise that strength. Your brain is the seat of *all* you feel, sense, experience; it is the seat of every last scrap of consciousness you possess or undergo; to get your brain—your intelligence—into high form and then to feel yourself using that quickened intelligence, that sharpened grasp . . . by all reports, it feels very, very good.

4
Improving Your Whole Brain, Physically

Your brain is a physical organ in your body.

Not many people will quarrel with that observation, or with the statement that your brain's functioning is affected by physical conditions and processes.

Like any other physical part of your body, when your brain is physically well off, it works better. When it is physically hampered, it works poorly.

As stated earlier in this book, your brain is the seat of every scrap of consciousness, behavior, and experience that can be considered part of your intelligence. Improve the physical condition of your brain and you improve the way your brain works.

Let us not enter here the argument of whether there is a consciousness which survives dissolution of the brain, a soul or synergy pattern which survives our deaths. Statements of that sort, because they are too hard to prove or disprove, do not belong in a book based on scientific findings. But we must note that as long as our consciousness depends on and is attached to our living body, it is our brain on which it must depend; that brain is a physical organ like any other physical organ, and the way in which it works can be directly helped or hindered by physical conditions, processes, and other specific physical events.

This chapter will deal with how to improve the physical condition of your *whole* brain. The next few chapters will tell you how to improve the way various *areas* of your brain are functioning. Later chapters go into nonphysical methods to improve the way your brain functions, mainly methods which affect the way your cortex, the highest part of your brain, functions. However, these latter, cortical methods are valuable only if your brain is in good physical condition and the lower, foundation areas of your brain can support the workings of an alert cortex.

How does one improve the physical condition of his own brain? Hidden from us by the skull, the brain has long been a source of fascination and mystery in our culture—since long before the time when biologists and physiologists first began to get a clear understanding of some of its processes.

The brain is an amazing piece of tissue, and we don't understand everything about it yet. The heart, too, is an amazing piece of tissue—so even is a fingernail, and I doubt that we understand everything about even a fingernail yet.

But the brain, by its very complexity, is something very special. In this age of cornea transplants, kidney transplants, heart transplants, people have begun talking (whimsically, I hope) about brain transplants. But if you transplanted Mr. Jones's brain into Mr. Smith's head, who would go home with whose wife? A brain transplant would not be a *brain* transplant, it would be a *body* transplant. Your brain is *you,* in more ways than not.

The brain is a physical organ performing and running on physical processes, some of which are understood and some of which are not. Those that we understand give us the means to change and improve the physical condition and workings of that brain.

Your brain is the most active part of your body, other than your heart. One third of all the oxygen used in your whole body, and therefore one third of all the food energy burned up by your whole physical body, is used up by your brain. In turn, your brain monitors and controls every process going on in every part of your body.

All the food energy, nutrition, and oxygen which your

brain gets must reach it through the carotid arteries, as we noted in chapter 2. Once inside the skull, smaller and more numerous arteries branch out from the larger carotids until a fantastically intricate network of capillaries laces throughout the brain.

That blood-carrying network has to reach as many brain cells as possible as successfully as possible because cells which aren't well supplied by capillaries simply don't develop, even when a lot of stimulus is poured into them. From there those capillaries are gathered into small veins, gathered into larger veins, eventually into the pair of jugular veins which return the used blood to the heart for recirculation to the lungs, where it is recharged with fresh oxygen. Once you are thirty years old, chances are that your brain's circulatory system has already started its long retreat and 100,000 of your least-nourished brain cells die every day. If you are thirty years old or older, chances are that more than 200 of your brain cells have died since you first began reading this very chapter. Several million of your brain cells are on the verge of dying and will do so within the next week or so.

Of course you have approximately 10 billion brain cells, so this is not immediately a very noticeable loss. And most of the cells which are lost are the unused, undeveloped ones. Yet 100,000 a day adds up after a while until your brain is seriously impaired. And developed, more active cells are lost as the brain's circulatory system deteriorates.

But as noted in chapter 2, you can not only prevent that circulatory deterioration but also greatly expand and improve your brain's circulatory system. Most of those several million brain cells of yours now on the verge of dying need not do so; they can recover as you restore and rebuild your brain's circulatory system.

Not only can you keep nourishing all those brain cells of yours which are presently nourished, but you can also nourish a lot of cells you are not presently nourishing, including a lot of cells which you have never nourished before.

For these latter, though, simply building up your circulatory system is not enough. Your newly reached brain cells must start developing, to make their own demands on your circulatory system themselves. If they fail to do so, your newly enhanced circulatory system will quickly abandon them once your peak efforts at brain-building are over. This means that improving your brain's circulatory system must be done in tandem with other procedures, stated elsewhere in this book, for "turning on" and developing your brain cells, or much of your effort will be wasted. Though you will get *some* effect regardless, you get by far your best results if you jam most of your brain-improving efforts into a concentrated, all-at-once, three-week period.

A fair amount of regular healthy exercise improves circulation and brings more nutrition more quickly to all your tissues, including those of your brain. Swimming, especially hold-your-breath-type underwater swimming, and jogging may be the best forms of exercise from this general circulatory standpoint, though some of the activities for direct effect on the brain which we will suggest in the next two chapters also are healthy forms of physical exercise.

Even better than these in directly improving the brain's circulation, though, is the simple method described in chapter 2, masking. Though rebreathing your own breath in a paper bag does not greatly reduce your oxygen over that thirty seconds, it increases by many times the tiny amount of CO_2 in your bloodstream. This harmless extra CO_2 induces the carotid valves to open wide, letting more oxygen, food energy, and nutrition through to the brain. If you mask for a half minute every half hour for two to three weeks, you will have trained your carotid valves to remain much wider open. These wide-open valves will not only cause full use of your brain's present capillary network, but trigger some further development and extension of that capillary network. Over the past decade or so, Philadelphia's Institutes for the Achievement of Human Potential have come to regard masking as one of their most potent methods for improving the physical condition and functioning of human brains; some thousands of patients have used masking safely and with powerful effect.

Some food elements are closely associated with development

and extension of the capillaries and, if added as supplements to your diet during your three weeks of masking and brain-building, should make your efforts several times more effective.

In a classic experiment in the 1950s, Puente-Dominguez and R. Dominguez experimentally created heightened need for circulatory expansion in dogs' heart tissues by tying off a branch of the coronary artery. Some dogs received no special diet; other dogs were dosed daily with d-alpha tocopherol (vitamin E). Those dogs dosed with vitamin E showed good recovery and, upon dissection, were found to have rapidly and extensively expanded their circulatory systems, including proliferations of new capillaries to get around the experimental blocks. Those dogs without vitamin E dosage showed poor recovery and little if any compensatory development of their circulatory systems around the blocks. It was vitamin E, specifically, that enabled the circulatory system to expand and develop to meet the new demands made upon it. (Reported in the eighth issue of *Summary,* 1956.)

A host of other medical studies have confirmed this circulation-improving effect of vitamin E, both in laboratory animals and in humans. Many of these are cited in Shute's annotated bibliography;[1] some of these and others are mentioned in many texts on nutrition, including an excellent one by Roger J. Williams.[2] The evidence is abundant; daily doses of vitamin E while you "mask" and build your brain should greatly improve your brain's circulatory system much more than will masking alone, and to that degree further aid the improvement of your physical brain and the intelligence which that brain sustains.

So much has been claimed for vitamin E that the American medical profession now tends to look askance at that controversial vitamin, even though some European medical cir-

---

1. Shute, Evan, "The Current Status of Alpha Tocopherol in Cardiovascular Disease," in Bailey, Herbert, *Vitamin E: Your Key to a Healthy Heart* (New York: Arc Books, 1966).

2. Williams, Roger J., *Nutrition Against Disease* (New York: Bantam Books, Inc., 1973).

cles have wholly embraced vitamin E as a preventative and cure for heart attacks, a cure for circulatory problems and childlessness, and a preventative for birth defects, among a host of other effects. Though no medical physician, this writer has himself had occasion to cite elsewhere [3,4,5] other evidence that mothers ingesting vitamin E throughout pregnancy and at the onset of labor will prevent much of the usual brain damage in fetuses and newborns and result in significantly more intelligent children.

Though the controversy has generated strenuous efforts on the part of some to discredit advocates of vitamin E, several of its well-known and well-proven effects apparently have never been seriously contradicted. One of those effects is the one above: when the body needs to proliferate new capillaries, veins, and arteries, vitamin E aids this proliferation better than any other known food element. Thus the vitamin can significantly aid you in improving your brain's circulatory system and the physical condition of your brain.

The other uncontradicted effect is that the vitamin, an antioxidant, improves tissue use of oxygen.[6,7,8] Thus, adding this vitamin to your diet should enable your brain to get better use out of whatever blood supply and circulatory system is available to it at any given time. In both these respects, then, vitamin E is clearly indicated as a great aid in improving the physical condition of your brain.

---

3. Wenger, Win., *On Raising Human Intelligence* (Federalsburg, Maryland: MCM Press, 1971).

4. ——— issue #3 of the *TRAHI Report: Newsletter of the Team for Research in Augmenting Human Intelligence,* 1971.

5. ——— "Intelligence and Vitamin E," *MENSA Bulletin* #148, September, 1971.

6. *Taber's Cyclopedic Medical Dictionary* (ninth edition, 1963).

7. Darlington, F. G. and Chassels, J. B., "Final, Inclusive Report on Five-Year Study on the Effects of Administering Alpha Tocopherol to Thoroughbreds," *Summary,* XII, 1960.

8. See also long list of studies, domestic and foreign, cited in Shute, *op. cit.*

Further, even those who most strenuously seek to discredit use of vitamin E admit that it is at least safe and harmless. (There are two exceptions to this harmlessness, however. First, diabetics, whose insulin need is reduced by the vitamin, must recalibrate their dosages or risk insulin shock. Second, though the vitamin is often used to lower high blood pressure, a few high-blood-pressure patients, starting in with massive dosages, found that vitamin E so strongly increased the strength and efficiency of their heartbeat that their blood pressure temporarily went up instead of down until their circulatory systems could adjust.)

Humans frequently have been given 3,000 international units a day of vitamin E without the slightest ill effects, and there is no indication that ill effects could result even from dosages many times greater than that.

It is best to begin vitamin E dosage slowly and build up; otherwise much of the vitamin may be wasted. From what various researchers in the field have published, it would seem best to begin with 30 i.u. a day of d-alpha tocopherol, toward the end of or immediately after a meal. Starting this a month before your all-out three-week period of masking and brain-building would give you time gradually to build your dosage up to 200–400 i.u. per day by the time you were ready to begin. Regular, moderate exercise may help your body take up and use all of the vitamin without wasting it.

Taking vitamin E is as easy as masking; any drug store has it available for over-the-counter sale.

Vitamin E may be the best single vitamin for helping your brain's circulation develop, but all the other food elements are also involved, at least to some degree. Every physical process in the human body involves *every* vitamin.[9] It is merely the *quantities* of each vitamin needed which always change from process to process, from organ to organ, and from tissue to tissue. Well-balanced meals, perhaps with a broad-spectrum multivitamin supplement pill, are therefore a good idea during your three-week concentrated brain-build. In fact, such might be a good idea for you the rest of the time as well.

---

9. Williams, *op. cit.*

But among all the other food elements besides vitamin E associated with every physical process, these in particular have been indicated as playing an important role in capillary development: choline,[10] vitamin C, and C-associated bioflavonoids, balanced, of course, by the other B vitamins.[11] For these, no dosage-build-up time has been indicated; apparently you can begin supplementing your diet with these right at the start of or just prior to your three-week brain-build.

This combination of dietary supplements, by the time you start regular masking and your three-week brain-build, should be very helpful in building your brain's circulatory system and thus the physical condition of your entire brain.[12]

Vitamin E, 200–400 i.u. per day
Choline, 200–400 i.u. per day, together with 2–3 tablets of broad-spectrum B-vitamin Brewers' Yeast to prevent imbalances
Bioflavonoids, 200 i.u. per day
Vitamin C, ½ gram per day
A general multivitamin, such as Vitamin-Quota's "Enterra," rich in B-vitamins, or Walgreen's "Basic Nutrition Supplement No. 127"

You may, of course, get temporary brain-boosts out of various of the B-vitamins, notably choline, B-1, and B-12. The brain's entire functioning is based largely on various forms of various B-vitamins. No impulses could transfer from one brain cell to the next without cholinasterase, for example, which is derived from choline, as are most of the chemicals used in and around the links between functioning brain cells. Megadoses of the B-vitamins are often used to treat various disorders of the brain, but their effect is temporary. Once the megadosage ends, the disorder returns.

---

10. Davis, Adelle, *Let's Get Well* (New York: Harcourt, Brace and World, 1965).

11. A series of references cited in Davis, *op. cit.*

12. Suggestion, *not* prescription. These are all nonprescription, readily bought over the counter at drugstores everywhere.

For some special occasion, a test or a time when you have to solve difficult problems, you can get some extra brain-boost from a third to a half gram of each of the three B-vitamins mentioned above, perhaps also from glutamic acid, the protein in which many people are reputed to be deficient. Should you take any B-vitamins in concentration, it is important to accompany it with some other broad-spectrum B-supplement such as Brewers' Yeast tablets, for your concentrated dosage may cause your body to use up other B-vitamins more rapidly and therefore create an artificial shortage.

There is not much point, however, in getting only a *temporary* boost in your intelligence, so we do not recommend this procedure of megadosing B-vitamins.

Your brain, just as any other part of your body, cannot work at its best as long as *you* aren't in shape to work at *your* best. When you are slightly ill or out-of-sorts, a surprisingly large number of your brain circuits are tied up in monitoring and trying to regulate the condition, below the threshold of your awareness; these circuits, and the energy they are using, subtract from what your brain could be bringing to bear on what's before your attention. If you let yourself remain chronically far below par, your brain could acquire the habit of chronically conserving energy and thereby slowing down the activities of the thinking and relating portions of your brain. That habit, by itself, can subtract very greatly from what your intelligence would otherwise be.

Maintain, restore, or build your general physical health, and your brain will work better as well. Regular moderate exercise, good nutrition, and a good physical checkup by a physician are very important.

If you can find a physician who can and will check for such things, get your nutritional balances tested. Individual biochemical makeup is always unique.[13] And most people

13. Williams, Roger J., *Biochemical Individuality* (New York: John Wiley & Sons, 1956).

are badly undernourished in at least some specific food elements.[14] Often a person can improve his well-being, efficiency, and I.Q. very drastically just by discovering and correcting some nutritional deficiency. Deficiency of *any* food element costs you *some* of your intelligence.[15]

Perhaps it goes without saying, but protecting your brain from injury is also important to improving and maintaining the physical well-being of your whole brain. By injury we mean not only the obvious mechanical things, like football and boxing or the risks incurred by not using seatbelts in your car, but drugs and drinking. Both "hard" and "soft" drugs, even marijuana, have been frequently cited as producing varying degrees of brain damage; for thousands of years alcohol has been known to produce this effect. One good drinking bout usually will wipe out tens of millions of your brain cells in one swat. Please note: your brain is the highest end product of two billion years of sophisticated evolution on this planet. Your brain is unique; there is nothing else like it; it is invaluable; it is a mechanism by far more intricate and more capable than any and every machine man has yet designed or even dreamed of designing. Your brain is *you*. Please don't scramble it.

One last suggestion for improving the physical condition of your whole brain applies to you only if you frequently have ups and downs, very good days and days when you function very poorly—and/or have "blank" moments when your mind just seems to stop registering things for a second or so.

Chances are that these blank moments and these days when you function poorly will go away if you reduce your fluid intake by one fourth to one third (and cut out alcohol). If you don't have these problems, your fluid level is fine: don't change it.

Dr. Robert Doman, physician and researcher at Philadelphia's Institutes for the Achievement of Human Potential,

---

14. Williams, 1973, *op. cit.*

15. *Ibid.*

has rediscovered what Hippocrates discovered two thousand years ago: If you have these problems, your brain is too wet. If you keep your fluid level too high, you even run the risk of an epileptic fit—the brain's attempt to reduce fluids in your skull and body to a safe level.

If, unfortunately, you happen to be epileptic and have been placed on one of the mind-dulling medications for it—like so many hundreds of thousands of people who have had their minds dulled by drugs for everything from epilepsy to "hyper-activity"—please get your physician to contact Dr. Robert Doman at Philadelphia's Institutes to check out whether yours is one of the types of epilepsy involving excess fluid. At this writing, chances are very strong that your physician has never heard of this discovery.

Too much white sugar can also produce a pattern of intermittent bad days, lassitude, and fatigue. Cutting down or cutting out white sugar, and the foods and drinks which contain it in large quantities, should also boost your efficiency and well-being.

In any case, those things which detract from your general physical health also detract, directly or indirectly, from your intelligence—and correcting these things will aid your intelligence. And, above all, specifically putting and keeping your brain in good physical health will aid your intelligence, masking and vitamin E being perhaps the two most powerful means to build your brain's physical well-being.

Besides these general measures involving the entire physical brain, though, is another set of considerations requiring us to delve down to specific lower levels of the brain and work on each of these levels individually, as we will discuss in the next chapter.

5 Improving the Key Lower Regions of Your Brain

Watch a baby's eyes as he creeps about the floor on hands and knees.

As each hand moves forward in turn, his eyes focus on it —then on the other hand as it shoves forward, then on the first again, back and forth.

Hundreds of thousands of times.

By creeping around on the floor he is training his eyes to work together at arm's length—the distance at which he will later read and write, perform arts and crafts, build and manipulate tools.

As Dr. Glenn Doman observes, civilization itself was built at arm's length. As Raymond Dart's[1] Institute of Man observes from exploring primitive and advanced cultures, tribes whose infants crawl and creep around freely on floor or ground tend to have advanced cultures and technology, and some form of written language. Tribes which restrict their infants from crawling and creeping around remain very backward, have no writing, learn reading when taught but only

1. Physician Raymond C. Dart, early and notable discoverer of *Australopithecus,* an important "missing" link in man's line of evolutionary descent, directs the Institute of Man, one of Philadelphia's Institutes for the Achievement of Human Potential.

with the greatest difficulties, and literally cannot *see* within arm's length though there is nothing physically wrong with their eyes.

One close study of two Indian tribes living in similar economic and social circumstance in the same physical environment, and living so closely to each other that their reservations intertwined, showed that the physical, cultural, and mental (by more than 25 points I.Q., among other measures) advantages belonged to the tribe which let its infants crawl and creep freely.[2] Other as-yet unpublished studies by the Institute of Man in Philadelphia show the same effects among other societies.

Hundreds of thousands of times, the freely creeping infant practices and trains his visual brain circuits to focus his eyes together and work them together at arm's length. Because of this training, his eyes are comfortable later when focused at that distance. They can form and hold a single image together at that distance easily and comfortably, and they can work together and follow a common path easily without strain or fatigue.

But what if the person as an infant did not have this freedom to move around? What if, instead, as so many babies are these days, he was restricted to a playpen for a significant part of his waking hours each day?

How long can you read comfortably before you have to look up briefly to relieve your eyes?

If you are not completely comfortable reading for at least fifteen minutes at a stretch without once looking away from the page for however brief an instant, and your vision is otherwise normal, then chances are that you did not do enough hands-and-knees creeping when you were an infant—whether you were kept in a playpen, or whether you just didn't move around much.

(*Don't* force yourself to glue your eyes to the printed page

2. Misner, William D., "The Significance of Mobility in Early Childhood: Comparison in Two American Indian Cultures," *Human Potential,* Vol. 2, No. 1, 1969.

—that would just strain them worse and deepen the problem. If your eyes look up from the page often, they *need* to look up from the page often, however much this diminishes your powers of concentration and following of sophisticated arguments. *If* you find yourself reading more comfortably for longer uninterrupted stretches, *as a result of* other things you did which are suggested in this chapter and book, *that* is the correct way to extend your visual attention span.)

Many people are more unfortunate in this respect. At least you are reading—this book, and other things. A great many American adults never read a book once they are out of school. According to Harvard studies, more than half of all American adults are too illiterate to read a daily newspaper. More than one third of all American schoolchildren, a percentage that is rising, regardless of whether they are taught reading by phonics, whole-word look-say, programming, or any other method when they enter school, are condemned to a lifelong reading disability. That disability need not be lifelong—but it will be, because most of America's educators, psychologists, and reading specialists refuse to treat the problem, the neurological problem, and only treat the symptoms (like a fireman blowing away the smoke instead of dousing the blaze).

If a reading-disabled person can't bring his eyes together to form a single image—if one eye looks at the start of a sentence and the other eye is halfway back up the page—what possible good can it do to tell the victim to sound out his ABCs?

And if you "correct" his eyes with glasses or surgery so that they point at the same place on the arm's-length printed page, those eyes still don't know how to work together. And they will be further than ever from learning how, for with such "correction" they are now being fed distorted information about what they are looking at. Only when the brain controlling those eyes is fed the correct, crucial information—the kind of information which that freely creeping infant practiced feeding into his young, pliant, growing brain hundreds of thousands of times—will those eyes learn to work together comfortably.

There is far more to be said on this point than this book, or any ten books, can adequately describe. Let us merely say here that the sense of sight handles more information than all other senses put together and thus involves most of your brain, the seat of your intelligence and organ of all your awareness and consciousness.

Let us merely say here that *you* can tell, from walking about the streets and shops, which children have been kept in playpens and which have not (adults' faces are more complicated, but sometimes you can tell there too). You can see it in their eyes.

Playpen eyes.

With your attention once drawn to this, you now have the inescapable tragedy of *knowing,* of being able to predict which children will have to suffer lifelong reading disabilities.

You know which ones as you see them around the neighborhood or in the streets and shopping centers. The dulled eyes, or the bright brassy stare, or the uninterested eyes, or the vague unfocused stare, or even the alert eyes that are still somehow "off," or the eyes out of which *not much* is looking on the world.

What has this discourse on children and playpens have to do with you, an adult? Your reading must not have been injured too badly or you would not be reading this book. But chances are that you were kept for *some* periods of time in a playpen, or that a brain injury before and/or during birth kept you from moving around as a baby as much as was needed, or that you were too swaddled in clothing most of the time to move around much. You can read, but chances are that you cannot read as well or as comfortably or with as unfettered attention as you could, had the vision circuits in your brain received full stimulus for development.

It is even possible that as an infant you might have been, for natural, hormonal reasons, naturally too passive and not moved around much—and this in itself would have developmentally injured your brain. In the extreme case of infantile passivity, those lovably placid Down's Syndrome victims often known as "Mongoloid idiots," it turns out that "Mongoloids'" brains are potentially okay, that it is their extremely placid nature which keeps them from moving and developing. More and more, Down's Syndrome patients have as infants been placed on programs of intensive sensori-motor exercise and other procedures devised by the Domans and Delacato at Philadelphia's Institutes for the Achievement of Human Potential. These infants, in Philadelphia and Brazil, are growing up with average intelligence and respiratory health and without the overt "Mongoloid" features we used to think were part of the unchangeable nature of Down's Syndrome victims. Several former Down's Syndrome patients, treated in the 1950s by other procedures which had the same sensori-motor galvanizing effect, are now reportedly attending college.

Why *is* infantile movement so vital to vision and intelligence?[3] For most of this century the basic facts have been well established on what "turns on" the brain and the cells and circuits within the brain—stimulus. Brain cells simply do not develop without stimulus. In 1911 one of the great brain histologists of all time, Ramon y Cajal,[4] published the results

---

3. Incidentally, you can protect your own children from the effects of too little movement. As soon as possible, even on the day of birth itself, induce your baby to start crawling around (crawling stomach-to-floor). Give him plenty of space to crawl in and a surface suitable for crawling. If he must wear clothing, his crawling surface must be smooth enough not to friction against those clothes—better to keep the house a few degrees warmer and let him go naked. By having him crawl, however slowly at first, to highly desired breast or bottle, or heading him down a long inclined plane so that his various movements translate into forward motion, or by the best method, tickling the sole of each foot in alternation, you can make even the most passive newborn used to moving around and encountering his environment. (For why foot-tickling is the best method, see further discussion in Wenger, Win, *On Raising Human Intelligence* [Federalsburg, Md.: MCM Press, 1971].)

4. Some of Ramon y Cajal's untranslated work is described by José M. R. Delgado in his *Physical Control of the Mind: Toward a Psycho-Civilized Society* (New York: Harper and Row, 1969).

of his previous thirty years' research, during which he found:

1) Not only stimulus, but especially stimulus in the form of feedback through the senses of effects produced on one's own perceptions of his environment by his own activities (including effects on that environment) is what develops the brain.

2) Of this sensory feedback, it is the feedback from the activities of infancy[5] that, by far, most develops the brain.

Astonishingly, nearly everyone overlooked these most important of all the findings this renowned pioneer of the brain made—or perhaps we'd all be geniuses today. It was not until the 1950s that Glenn and Robert Doman and Carl Delacato, under the tutelage of the renowned Temple Fay, independently rediscovered much the same findings as those made by Ramon y Cajal and developed a working cure for mental retardation, brain damage, cerebral palsy, and reading and speech disabilities, built partly around the infantile activities of creeping and crawling. Like so many of the other contributors to human health and well-being, in the mid 1960s the Doman-Delacato approach came under furious attack and was nearly driven out of existence as funding dried up. But that approach, and the institutes themselves, stood up successfully under the brunt of those attacks, were thoroughly vindicated, and as this book is written are coming back into standing, however painfully, among professionals in medicine and education.[6]

5. For reasons which are perfectly evident, biologically.

6. As the overt errors of the attacks became evident, two of the attacking paraprofessional organizations retracted immediately and a third of the six did so later. A fourth launched into an antagonistic study which, to its chagrin, so verified the few elements of Doman-Delacato procedure it tested that in 1973 it was preparing publication of those results with a retraction of its role in the attacks. Further discussion of these attacks may be found in Wenger, *op. cit.,* but the full story, with all its elements and involvements and strange implications, has not yet unfolded and is worthy of a book in itself by some capable historian—or by a detective.

The point for us to note here is that both these independent discoverers, Ramon y Cajal and Fay-Doman-Delacato, found that the most effective way to develop the brain is to give it the sensory feedback from infantile sensori-motor activities.

To grasp this key point in depth, let's take a quick look at the brain. When the earth was inhabited largely by fish, all the brain they needed was the spinal cord and medulla, which control heartbeat, respiration, and other basic body processes, but register only the most primitive sensory experiences and provide only the most primitive motor activities. That cord and medulla, first brain and fish brain, are all the newborn baby really has working once he has come out of his fishlike existence in the sea of the womb. All other levels of his brain have to be developed, by experience.

Atop the medulla and cord sits the pons, that portion of our brain which was developed by the first land animals. Where the medulla registers sense impressions most primitively, reacting to alternation only (changes in light and dark and color, in sound level, in tactile/touch impression, etc.), the pons handles sense inputs at a much more sophisticated level. This pons can manage the trick of perceiving differences in light value within the same visual field—i.e., it can see outlines. The pons can perceive some basic elements and patterns in sound and touch and other senses. For reasons imposed on it much later in evolution, in the earliest days of the most primitive mammals whose live-born young had to make it to the milk line or pouch to hang on and survive, the pons has a precocious ability to bring its motor function into play at birth—crawling, stomach-to-floor. If not encouraged to crawl when most ready, the human infant may miss the crawling stage altogether, going on much later to hands-and-knees creeping, thus leaving his pons poorly developed and handicapping to some degree all his later development.

Like a great hand closing over the tiny fist of medulla and pons is the midbrain, first developed by the reptiles. Competition on land, at that stage of our evolution, had gotten a lot tougher, and to capture prey or to escape being preyed upon, the reptiles found it dangerously slow going to continue sliding around on their bellies. Except for snakes, a much later development, reptiles mastered the third dimension, the vertical, getting up to totter around and, eventually, to run around on all fours.

This third, spatial, upright dimension requires a wholly greater order of magnitude of sensori-motor development, including mastery of that intricate web of perceptions linked to the art of balancing in the upright. Thus, the midbrain has to be many times larger than the medulla, cord, and pons put together. The senses are greatly more sophisticated—to the point where many, many even tiny differences in light value can be seen within the same visual field: the midbrain can make out details within those outlines that the pons sees, a logical progression in which each brain level learns and compounds its seeing from what the level beneath it saw. Pattern and detail recognition in the other senses is similarly sophisticated in the midbrain. Except for the much later developments of swinging from overhead branch or handhold to branch and of upright walking on the hind legs, most physical coordination is learned at the midbrain level.

As every schoolboy knows (except for several states where it is *still* illegal to teach about evolution), our reptilian ancestors became mammals. At this time, the cortex was developed, a much larger hand enclosing the midbrain hand wrapped around the tiny fist of pons and medulla. Certain rather ratty mammals couldn't make out very well on the dangerous ground and took first to the bush, then to the trees, and became monkeys. Some of these tree swingers did very well and became many and large—and then, either they got crowded out of the trees by their own numbers, or the climate turned drier and reduced their treeland habitat. Whichever happened (and evidence suggests that both did), those poor tree-swinging ancestors of ours were robbed of their trees. Willy-nilly, they were forced down to the dangerous grasslands and streams to become apes. And, probably from the same background of the ground apes, man evolved.

This rapid-fire series of evolutionary challenges created a biological freak—the human cortex, capable of adapting its creature to almost *anything*. The demands placed on that cortex are so many and so drastic and so varied that 90 percent of all human brain cells are in the cortex. It is with the cortex that we speak, think, walk, run, marvel at beauty, love (with twongs from our medulla), scheme and hate, contemplate microbes and galaxies, destroy and replant forests and fields and cities and civilizations, and experience the sense of wonder.

This freakish cortex of ours has given us the means to free ourselves of further evolutionary necessity (instead of growing a set of wings in a few hundred thousand years, we can build an airplane immediately) and to figure our way out of almost any problem. Unfortunately, our cortices are poorly developed in most instances, and this has been true for most of us ever since we found a way to build the first civilizations and discovered: easy living; slavery; routine and boredom; drudgery; confinement of all sorts; mercy for the less fortunate; welfare programs; pollution; and so on.

Just before the dawn of civilization, Cro Magnon man was a physical masterpiece, able to run down rabbit and deer on foot. Cro Magnon was an artistic giant; the sophistication of his cave paintings still excites wonder. He was a mental giant, building from scratch the bases of the first civilizations before his culture had the technical and scientific awarenesses which would have made the task feasible. Take a pure Cro Magnon and place him among us today, let him assimilate the richly simplifying awarenesses of our science, art, and culture—and he would surpass Newton, Einstein, and Leonardo.

Our brains are 15 percent smaller than the brain of our Cro Magnon ancestor. Nearly all the loss is in that freakish cortex; most of that loss is in the most advanced, highest regions of that cortex. If evolutionary history repeats itself as it has with other species, loss of that much of our most adaptive feature, the human cortex, could even foreshadow eventual extinction of the human species. What we have lost from that wonderful Cro Magnon brain represents unimaginable, irreplaceable realms and possibilities. But that shrunken and tattered remnant of human cortex that remains is still capable of almost anything—if we develop it well.

Our environment is full of stimuli: signs, periodicals, radios, and TV bombard us with information; our civilization has amassed an incredible wealth of understanding-on-tap. Why, *why* are our cortices so poorly developed?

The answer is in the structure of the brain and the way it develops. In keeping with so many other models of human development devised in many different sciences, let us picture the brain's structure and development as organized by stages. Development of one stage is prerequisite for development of the next, higher stage. Lower stages are more limited; higher stages enjoy more possibilities and scope. Rich developing of one stage allows the next stage to develop richly and well; poor development of or injury to one stage means that the next stage (and, consequently, all higher stages) can only develop poorly. Such maldevelopment at one level produces a "hangup" which warps and cripples all higher stages. In matters of brain structure, as in so many other models of human development, cure of maldevelopment at higher stages depends on reaching the lower-level deficiencies, feeding in enough experience at this lower level to bridge those deficiencies, and then pouring in more experience at successively higher levels to make up their deficiencies in turn. The reason that our information-rich environment doesn't better develop our cortices is that our lower brain levels are poorly developed.

To greatly simplify our picture of the brain, let us show it, as in figure 1, as an upside-down pyramid balanced on the spinal cord. Each level is essential to development of the next, higher level; each level enjoys a full order of magnitude of capabilities, experiences, functions, and possibilities greater than the level beneath, which "tutored" it.

In figure 2 we've compared this "standard" model to the model of scope of brain functions and experiences resulting from damage to or poor development of a lower level, and to the greatly expanded model of higher development proceeding from enrichment of lower levels. If indeed there is any limit to how far that higher development can go, no one has yet discovered it.

To date there is much less data on the repair and enrichment of adult brains than on the repair and enrichment of

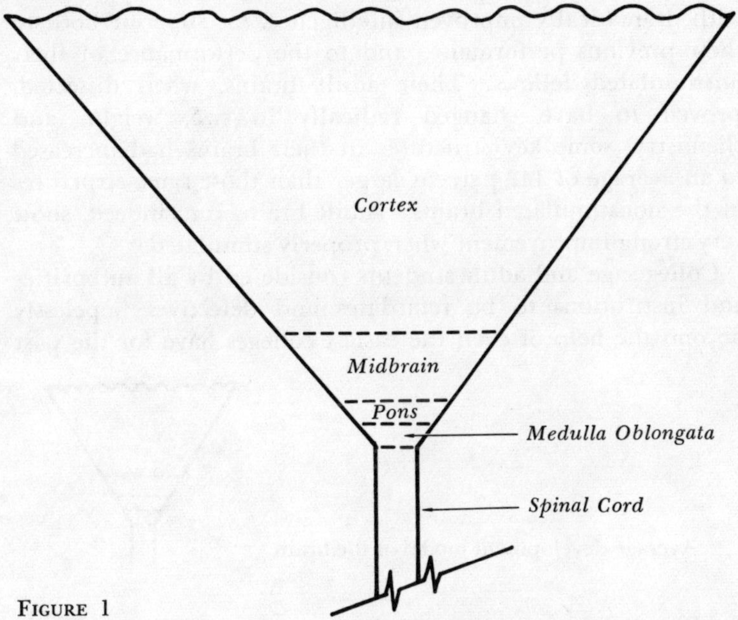

FIGURE 1

children's brains. This is because the originators and principal practitioners of the method that works best so far—the still-developing Doman-Delacato procedures—are emotionally and deeply committed to putting all their scarce resources into improving the well-being of children, who have more of their lives yet to live than older people do, and who are easier to change.

But adult and even aged brains also respond well to the Doman-Delacato procedures and other enrichments. In the most concrete demonstrations, the indefatigable Altman and Das, oftentime colleagues of the even more indefatigable David Krech, suddenly subjected *adult* laboratory animals to a radically more stimulating environment for a few weeks, then tested their abilities in comparison with litter-mates not so stimulated. Altman and Das then sacrificed and physically dissected these adult animals to look for physical changes in the brain.

After stimulation, those *adult* laboratory animals performed with dramatically improved intelligence, far superior both to their previous performance and to the performance of their unstimulated fellows. Their adult brains, when dissected, proved to have changed radically in size, weight, and chemistry; some key structures in their brains had increased to an average of 142 percent larger than those same structures in the nonstimulated brains.[7] Adult brains can, indeed, show very strong improvement when properly stimulated.

College-age and adult students considered by all authorities and institutions to be retardates and defectives hopelessly beyond the help of even the easiest colleges have for the past

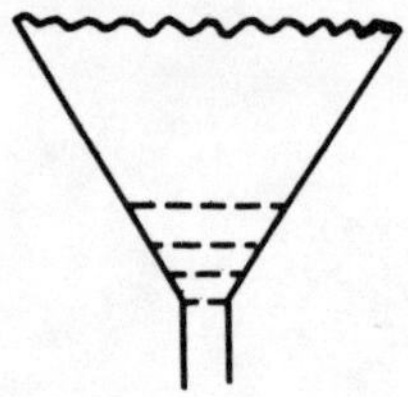

Average development model of the brain.

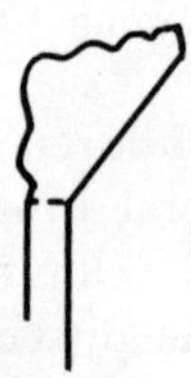

Deficient development. Put in experience to enrich and rebuild lower levels, or the higher levels cannot develop properly.

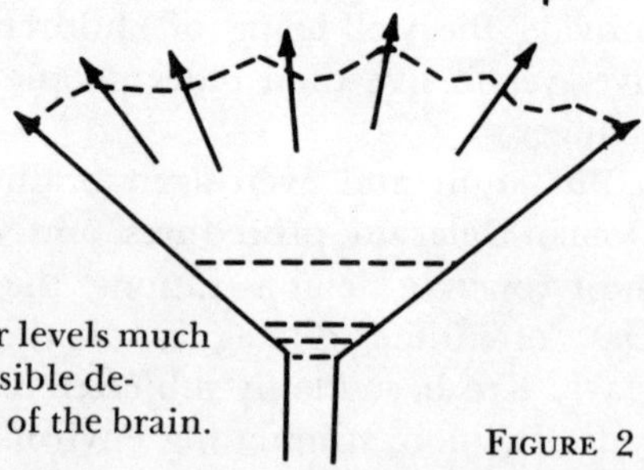

Better enrichment of lower levels much improves the range for possible development of higher levels of the brain.

FIGURE 2

7. Altman, Joseph and Das, Gopal D., "Autoradiographic Examination of the Effects of Enriched Environment on the Rate of Glial Multiplication in the Adult Rat Brain," *Nature,* Vol. 204, 1964.

eight years been sought out and treated with Doman-Delacato procedures at Plano Development Center, just north of Dallas, Texas. Half of these deficient learners have been so improved as to be able to move on successfully into a standard liberal-arts program at another college, according to Dr. Robert Morris, chancellor of the University of Plano. Some of these once-deficient learners are now in graduate studies.

The more developed—the more adult, if you prefer—a brain is, the more receptive it is to stimulus and the more it does with that stimulus. But the adult brain is also more stabilized, and stability resists change. Many adults are also often more self-conscious and thus may balk at doing such things as masking or practicing hands-and-knees creeping—even in the secure privacy of their own homes. Letting that angel with the flaming sword of self-consciousness bar you from your personal Eden of self-development seems silly and trivial, but it often happens.

And you may give that self-consciousness a bit of a workout during the three weeks you spend pouring in enough concentrated stimulus to shift that stability of your adult brain. For, as we have seen in this chapter, it is the feedback through the senses from activities of infancy which most stimulate the brain to develop. It is the first three brain sections of infancy—medulla, pons, and midbrain—whose levels of experience must be revisited and reenacted, awakened and enriched, if we are later to improve successfully our levels of cortical intelligence.

"Except ye become as little babes, ye shall not enter . . ."

6
At the Foundations of Your Brain

Alternation. Light and dark and shift of color. Primitive motion. Warm and cool. Pressures and release of pressures. These are the experiences of your medulla, the pivotal foundation of that upside-down pyramid which is your brain.

Have you ever hung underwater, either with scuba gear or on a hold-your-breath basis, and just let impressions flood into you? In large part you are revisiting the level of experience of the medulla—in more ways than one, for that medulla was the only working brain of fish.

Have you ever been very drunk, so that all that came to you were intermittent, raw, stark, basic sensations and impressions? I hope you haven't been, since alcohol and particularly drunkenness are tremendous damagers of the brain. But if you have been and can recollect such a state, you underwent this medullalike experience because you had intoxicated and knocked out all higher levels of the brain. A close call for you, because if that alcohol had penetrated to and deranged your medulla as well, which governs your heart, breath, and all other processes of your body, you'd be dead.

Alternation. Impressions register, then go away or shift to some other impression. That is life as a medulla creature.

Obtain access to some suitable body of water or a fair-sized swimming pool—municipal, school, YMCA, country club, or whatever. During your three-week brain-boosting marathon, each day spend at least a half hour "hanging" or floating stably deep under water and also atop the water in a face-down position, a completely relaxed "dead man's float." Don't use scuba gear. Stay under water for one, two, even three minutes at a time as your wind improves, on a hold-your-breath basis—you will be getting double benefit from this. Not only will you be adding experience at the level of your medulla, you will get the same benefit as in masking, that is, CO_2-training the valves in your carotid arteries to let more oxygen and nutrition through to your brain.

In the same pool, also on a hold-your-breath-under-water basis, swim actively for a total of fifteen minutes per day, both with vigorous underwater swim strokes and the more casual moving around under water. Let all your sensations come flooding in, and enjoy them as much as possible. Pleasure sensitizes, so the more you come to enjoy this underwater medulla existence, the more medulla-developing sensation you will derive from it.

Back home, re-create more of this alternating-impressions-type world for your medulla. Purchase a string or two of flashing Christmas-tree lights, string them up in various patterns at various distances from your chair in a quiet room to which you will go for a half hour at late twilight or at night to rest and relax.[1] A simple flasher for a regular lamp is not a bad idea either, provided it is only one of several light sources in the room.

In the daytime on sunny days, fill flat pans with water and prop them outside on sunlit windowsills or on the ground where wind and sun will catch them and reflect dancing light on the ceiling inside. This can be part of the visual backdrop for your other activities during the daytime.

Although the changes in their light intensity are slow and

1. The same arrangement of Christmas-tree lights, flashing around a newborn's crib for an hour an evening during his first one and one half to two weeks of life, will aid that infant's vision and subsequent intelligence to an extraordinary extent.

therefore of reduced value, the wealth of color, intensity, pleasure, and scope of sunrise and sunset probably make these of some value to your medulla. It would not hurt to take in a few of these during your three-week brain-boosting, and at other times as well.

Here is a trick of visual intensification which probably will help your medulla as well as other parts of your brain. When among other people, for several minutes at a time (totaling fifteen minutes to a half hour daily) flick your gaze from face to face, not letting your gaze rest on any one face for more than a half second at a time. When traveling or moving about, do the same thing with various features of the landscape or cityscape through which you are moving. Rig up one room in your house with pictures and many highly varied objects of visual interest and flick your gaze around these.

Your eyes perform the odd trick of registering far more information in the first instant of looking at something than at any other time. In fact, if you look at anything fixedly enough for long enough, you can no longer see it until you move your eyes. So—*flick*—looking—*flick*—every half second —*flick*—at a different—*flick*—visual object will pour far more visual information into your brain than usual, and thus begin to stretch and improve your brain's information-handling capacity.

Something as ordinary as increasing your vitamin A intake improves the ease, speed, and sensitivity of detail with which your eyes pass on information to your brain. Pilots of bombers on night missions used to swallow 200,000 international units or more of vitamin A to better see what they were doing. (Doctors recommend a safe maximum of 20,000 i.u. Unlike vitamin E, you *can* get too much vitamin A—it will bring on headaches—but most people would have to cram in 100,000 i.u. a day for weeks to reach that point. Moreover, discomfort or ill effects of excess vitamin A can be quickly corrected by about a half gram of vitamin C, which is partly antagonistic to A.) Twenty thousand i.u. a day of vitamin A, by improving your eyes' input to the brain, could help your brain develop if you are already giving that brain a pretty good workout on other counts, especially during your three-week brain-boosting marathon. Check with your physician if you are in doubt about dosage.

Lay out and glue onto some surface alternating strips of sandpaper, velvet, and other textures. Feel these, after dark or with eyes closed—the sense of touch is important to the lower levels of your brain. With eyes shut or the room dark, move around and feel the various textures and objects without trying to identify them—feel the feeling, not the object, so to speak.

Feel some touch-interesting object each day and study, by sight and feel, the hand with which you are doing the touching.

Open a succession of spices and condiments, give each a one-second sniff, then go back and linger over those which most please you. Again, don't identify them at this medulla stage, merely take in the sensation of their different odors.

Underwater swimming also provides medulla-level hearing experience. Other sources of such experience are: sit next to a secretary while she is typing, or a worker hammering, or a dripping faucet. Drop a ball, then close your eyes and listen to it bounce. A pendulum clock. Listen to your own heartbeat. Rhythm soothes. As fetuses we all listened to our mothers' heartbeats for crucial, growing months, even to the point where newly weaned puppies are quieted by a ticking alarm clock and human babies frequently prefer being held on the mother's left side.

Oddly enough, a motor activity in the pons, a higher level of the brain, proves to be crucial to further development of the medulla. Crawling stomach-to-floor, as the head turns from side to side, provides alternation in the senses of sight, sound, touch, and position. More important, crawling provides this alternation as feedback from the total sensori-motor gestalt, or pattern, of an infantlike activity—as Ramon y Cajal has taught us, this makes crawling a most powerful brain developer.

You should do a half hour to a full hour's worth of stomach-to-floor crawling every day during your three-week brain-boost, broken up into five- to ten-minute sessions scattered throughout the day. For some people this is the hardest step in brain-building.

Crawling is a most inefficient method of moving around. It seems, to say the least, undignified. And for the people who need it most—those who as babies never or rarely got to crawl around—it feels particularly awkward and difficult. No matter how awkward and difficult crawling feels to you, learning it and practicing it is crucial to the development of your brain—a missed stage, a missing link in the networks of your brain.

Don't worry about style, about "doing it right." If you follow some instruction or formula for crawling correctly, you will teach your cortex instead of your pons how to crawl—and this is of no benefit to you. If you don't know how to start, lie there stomach-down on the floor and, *without* lifting off the floor, simply *move* forward a few inches. Move forward any old way; just make sure that your stomach remains in contact with the floor. With enough practice, you'll find a more comfortable and effective way to crawl stomach-to-floor. This is the way to make sure that your pons, and not your cortex, is what learns to crawl. Your cortex can learn anything and is not the limiting factor in your brain's development. So crawl with your pons; don't think about your crawling posture, do it *without* cortical thought.[2] Crawling is one of the few things the pons can learn, and it *is* a very limiting factor in your brain's development.

In contrast to the other methods described in this chapter for "turning on" the foundations of your brain, crawling is hard work. The other methods are placid, restful, relaxing—

---

2. One of several flaws in a study by M. P. Robbins, which served as basis for the aforementioned attacks on Doman-Delacato procedures, was that instead of the Doman-Delacato procedures purportedly tested, Robbins taught the forms of crawling and creeping cortically to his subjects, so that their gains were insignificant. If after you've pons-learned crawling and practiced it awhile you want to make sure you have it correct, you can check yourself against the descriptions of crawling in Delacato, Carl, *A New Start for the Child with Reading Problems: A Manual for Parents* (New York: David McKay Co., 1970).

but crawling is probably the hardest work you will have to do throughout your three-week brain-building marathon. But watch an infant struggling to crawl—it's hard work for him, even harder than it is for you. But his desperate, repeated, sustained, all-out effort to crawl is a vital part of his human development. Your own not-so-difficult-but-still-hard work on this point is a vital part of your becoming a better human being.

7 Developing Your Second Brain—the Pons

It was from your medulla's experience of alternating light values that your pons learned to see simultaneous differences in light value in the same visual field—in other words, to see profiles and outlines. It was your medulla's experience of shifting impressions in each of your other senses that taught your pons to sense recognizable patterns in sound, touch, taste, smell, position, and combinations of these. Among the combinations, of special import to human beings is the medulla's accumulation of visual, touch, and position impressions that first enabled the pons to begin tracking both eyes together on the hand or on other moving objects.

The pons is the deepest level to which significant brain damage usually extends, because if that damage were to afflict the medulla, which controls our body's vital processes, it would derange those processes and we would die. Usually the pons is less vulnerable to injury, and less injured, than the midbrain, which in turn is much less injured and injurable than is the cortex (but the cortex is far more flexible in the methods by which it can learn and develop), so that by and large most of the deficiencies in our pons are usually deficiencies of development stemming from our being too constricted and understimulated as infants. Whatever the origin of our pons deficiencies, it is now our task to manipulate sense-inputs in such a way as to open up new brain-cell circuits in that pons.

Again, as at other brain levels, vision looms large in the development of the pons. Crawling, which links the left hand to the left eye and the right hand to the right eye, is essential to the pons as well as to the medulla. Underscore crawling, then, as an activity for pons development. The recommended amount of time, as noted before, is a half hour to an hour a day for three weeks.

Did you know that as far as the sides of your vision are concerned, your brain is an idiot? Looking straight ahead at some fixed point without letting your eyes stray to the side, place your hand about forty-five to seventy degrees from your center line of vision, but where you can still see it. Hold up several fingers. There they are, in your field of vision—now, by sight, count those fingers!

Surprised? Don't be too surprised by your inability to count one, two or three fingers at the sides of your field of vision. Just as you'd much rather walk than crawl or creep because it's easier, your brain would rather pay attention to only the very center of your field of vision because that, too, is easier.

Your brain receives impressions from the sides of your vision, but it doesn't do anything with those impressions—thus, those portions of your brain which receive those vision-edge impressions remain at an idiot level of intelligence. They are not linked into the more complex networks of your brain, so they cannot draw on those networks to interpret the impressions they have received—thus, you can't even count the number of fingers in plain sight! More important, those vision's-edge sections of your brain, by not being linked into your more complex networks, *are not contributing anything to the workings of those more complex brain networks!*

But those portions of your brain are not idiot by nature; they are idiot by default. You can easily train them and, in so doing, link them into the more complex processing networks of your brain. Once linked in, with time these once-idiot portions of your brain should gradually start contributing more to the operations of those networks, cumulatively raising your over-all intelligence long after your training has finished.

One lesson which has come through loud and clear in all the research done on the brain during the past few decades is this: When you improve the ability of any one part of the brain, you improve, at least to some extent, the functioning ability of the entire brain. Even the simplest brain circuits involve thousands of interlinked brain cells lacing through in sometimes unexpected directions. Most circuits link millions of cells, lacing through all areas and levels of the brain. Add to those circuits and you add to the range and complexity of functions they can perform.

How can you train the side-vision areas of your brain? First, mark a point on the far wall across from you and rivet your eyes onto it, resisting that urge to "sneak a peek" sideways.

Clicking a pencil flashlight on and off, test all around the edges of your field of vision to see in which sectors you see the light most clearly, and in which you see it least clearly. If you cannot see the blinking light fairly clearly at an angle of seventy to eighty degrees from the center of your vision, you should begin work with your medulla first. Break out those flashing Christmas-tree lights again and arrange them in a circle around a point on the wall eighty degrees from your line of vision to the first point. Through twelve to twenty five-minute sessions spaced over two to three days, with your eyes on the first point, pay attention to each flashing Christmas-tree light in turn and identify its color.

Make a set of highly distinctive cutouts, black on white or vice versa—a square, triangle, circle, crescent, irregular, and so on. Make the figures a foot high—later make similar figures six inches high, yet others three inches. Now you are ready to train your pons to see out of the corners of your eyes.

At the point farthest from your center of vision at which you can identify the figures, practice identifying them. Pick them up one at a time without looking directly at them, and identify them. See how far and how fast you can extend the range at which you can make these identifications.

This is an easy way to "turn on" new brain circuits in great quantity, but it consumes unexpectedly large amounts of energy. At first you will find this procedure physically tiring, so break it up into very short, very frequent practice sessions—perhaps three minutes every half hour.

With enough practice you should be able to identify increasingly smaller figures more and more easily and quickly at greater angles from your center of vision—and it will become less tiring. You will have "turned on" and linked in great swaths of your brain cells.

Similarly, to train your vision's edge in midbrain and cortex, repeat this procedure with more and more complexly detailed objects, with subtler distinctions. Again, repeat the procedure for counting numbers of fingers or objects held up.

By the same method you can even teach the side-vision areas of your brain to read!

One limitation: No matter how well you train the side-vision areas of your brain, the sides of your vision will always remain coarser than the center—this is not the fault of the brain but of the eye itself and so cannot be overcome by training. But even so, you should become able to read, count, and make out and identify fairly fine detail at seventy to eighty degrees from your line of vision all around—and the impact of this new ability on the rest of your brain will be unmistakable. Over a period of time, weeks and years after this three-week brain-boosting marathon, you will find your mind noticing more things, doing more things, performing feats which earlier would have astonished you.

Self-training in tasks of speed might be advisable, in view of the more complex things your more complex brain circuits are doing. But in most instances this more complex brain will actually speed up its operations, not slow them down, with all the added circuitry and perceptions.

Important to the pons, as noted at the beginning of this chapter in connection with crawling, is "bonding" or coordinating the left eye with the left hand and the right eye with the right hand. You can reinforce this bonding far beyond the limits of crawling. Perform one-handed tasks of manipulation at the extreme edges of your vision—putting a pencil through a ring, tracing out a maze, typing, dialing a phone, drawing pictures, putting your finger on a target, opening a can, playing chess or tennis or ping-pong. Practice these things, left hand at seventy to eighty degrees from the center of vision of your left eye, right hand similarly distanced from the center of vision of your right eye—and you will be well on the way toward developing a strong pons, which is the basis for enriching the development of all the rest of your brain.[1]

---

1. While most other procedures cited herein derive from other sources and researchers, this approach using side-vision areas of the brain appears original with this writer. The discovery is so recent that we don't yet know by how much or how rapidly this approach raises intelligence, but that it has this effect appears unmistakable. Within that approach, the progression from flashing colored lights and stark cutouts to finely detailed pictures and objects is derived from Doman-Delacato theory.

8
More Pons, Plus

So far in discussing your second brain, the amphibian pons, we have dealt only with vision, and almost exclusively with side vision. However major the effects of side-vision training on eventual intelligence, let us not forget to enrich your pons in other aspects as well—all improvements at pons level are important to the rest of your brain.

If you can borrow a tachistoscope from some school, your next step in training should be very easy. If you cannot obtain a tachistoscope, substitute an ordinary slide projector with a hand-held screen blocking the lens for all but an instant. If you cannot obtain either tachistoscope or slide projector, have a partner hold up objects and flashcards. Without tachistoscope, projector, or partner, arrange two mirrors facing each other to give you distance sighting on objects and on flashcards you hold in your hand (in this last instance, arrange strong lighting on where you will hold those objects and flashcards).

First with outlines (pons-level seeing). Proceed from larger to smaller figures, from one at a time to as many at a time as you can identify, from sharp contrasts to subtler and more difficult-to-see distinctions, from long gazes in which you can recognize everything to shorter and shorter instants in which to grasp the total scene at a glance (this is why the timed shutter of the tachistoscope would be handy). This is an exercise for center-line vision, even though it might parallel what you are doing with your edge-of-vision brain development.

At each point where identification becomes difficult for you, practice until those identifications are no longer difficult, and then move on to a new level of difficulty. Two to four twenty-minute sessions of such practice each day are probably best for you during your three-week brain-boosting marathon. If this proves tiring, you are probably "turning on" more brain cells than usual for this exercise: make your practice sessions shorter but much more frequent. There is no point of maximum difficulty; you can doubtless practice this kind of visual identification throughout your entire three weeks and beyond and still be making significant gains at the end.

The object of these exercises is to train your brain for more information input and handling, not to correct your probably nearsighted/farsighted/astigmatic vision. Without your glasses these exercises might produce a little such corrective effect, but if removing your glasses markedly slows down the rate at which visual information enters your brain during these exercises, keep your glasses on. These exercises would not correct your vision enough anyway to avoid wearing glasses afterward; though there are a few practitioners who use similar, sensori-motor exercises to correct over-all vision, these practitioners are as yet very few.

For enriching midbrain and cortex, follow the above procedures, but for more finely detailed pictures and objects rather than outlines.

For your sense of hearing at pons level and above, you can proceed to enrich both your sensitivity and ability to handle complexity.

Taking complexity first: This writer has the strong suspicion that a good recording of Johann Sebastian Bach's *Fifth Brandenburg Concerto* played on a high-quality stereo and listened to carefully two times a day throughout your three-week brain-boosting marathon, will immensely improve your hearing and make it more sophisticated. Chances are everything will sound different to you after this experience.

If music like this is definitely not your "bag," you can still sophisticate your hearing of speech. Acquire or obtain access to a quarter-track or two half-track tape recorders or cassettes. Record one conversation or line of speech, then overlay it with a second. Play back until you can follow both sets of talking at the same time. Repeat with two different sets of talking, and yet two others, until you can readily follow two simultaneous conversations. Now try it with three at a time. Loss of definition probably makes three your ceiling, though some individuals have been able to sophisticate their hearing to a point where they could follow four conversations simultaneously.

Sensitivity to sound is much easier still. One way is to pause every now and then and make note of everything you hear going on around you. At pons level, just listen to the sounds, however faint; at midbrain and cortex level, try to identify each—make a list on paper of everything you hear (not forgetting to include the sound of pen or pencil on paper), and try to extend that list during each session.

Another way to increase sensitivity to sound is to turn down the volume on radio or TV so that you can barely hear the talking—then follow that talking, and then turn down the sound a bit more—for ten to fifteen minutes a day. If you like music, play your very favorite pieces at virtually inaudible levels, and prepare to be surprised at how much you can actually pick up.

If you have a partner, have him or her make faint sounds for you to locate and identify. If not (or even if you do), go to unfamiliar places and see how much you can tell about each place just by the sounds you hear. As with other senses, the sensitivity to sound is more likely determined by your brain than by your ears, and so is readily improved by training such as we have just described.

To increase your sensitivity to smell, arrange your spices and condiments in some order of scent, and sniff through the sequence a few times. Change them to some other-patterned order and sniff through a few more times. Still at pons level, don't identify the scents, just smell them. At midbrain and cortical levels, see what you can identify by scent.

Although Western culture plays it down, touch is still very important to us. Taboos against touch upset us if we accidentally brush against a stranger on the sidewalk. The touch of a lover's hand or skin is almost unbearably pleasing. A child seeks reassurance by touch. Our language shows the importance of touch in its own way: we want to stay *in touch* with someone; someone else *rubs* us the wrong way; we want to get the *feel* of a given situation; John may be a *smooth* character but Jack is pretty *slick*.

In the dark or with eyes shut, continue the feeling of textures and household objects that you were doing to aid your medulla. Now arrange touch experiences in some sort of patterned sequence (as with the scents, above), rough/smooth/smooth/rough or some such, and explore the rhythm of tactile sensations—not just with your hands, but with your feet and other parts of your body as well.

As with scents, for pons-level touch don't identify, just *feel*. For midbrain and cortical touch, identify objects around the house, objects in a grab bag, denomination of coins in your pocket (a few people even reach a point where they are able to read the dates on their coins by touch). Practice differentiating, by touch, closely similar objects until you become sensitive to even the finest differences—again, you are not limited to your hands.

Near the top of the pons another visual skill becomes important, and becomes increasingly important and sophisticated as we ascend through midbrain and cortex: both eyes simultaneously tracking the same moving hand or moving object. This takes us into a different ball game.

9
Your Third Brain, Your Midbrain: Into the Third Dimension

Though the young infant should spend the majority of his time on his stomach, by the time he is well into pons development he can flip over onto his back, and so spends more and more time on his back. While he is on his back his natural motions repeatedly bring one or the other of his hands into full view and he begins to see them. The baby's delighted discovery of his own hands is a favorite scene for parents and photographers alike, and can be enriched and speeded by your making his hands easier for his eyes to find—such as giving him open-fingered, red-and-white striped "find-me mitts."[1]

Though that infant's problems are certainly not your problems, there is a connection. In this, as in so many other things, you did not complete the job that the infant started. Just as your brain got lazy and settled for interpreting your center of vision only; just as you prefer to walk because it is easier, even though crawling and creeping would remove bottlenecks holding back development of the rest of your mind; so also your brain developed hand-eye coordination only to the

1. Frequently such "find-me mitts" are supplied with such items as the first-level Playtentials sets developed by Harvard psychologist Burton White and produced by Kenner, Inc.

point that circumstances required of it, maybe a little beyond that point, and then gradually quit.

If time permits, and if you have a good player to practice against, during your marathon or at other times, table tennis is an excellent way to extend this hand-eye coordination. That game has many benefits: it demands very fast, complex reactions; you get instant feedback on your responses; the game has many subtleties, finesses, interlinked skills, rhythms, and stratagems which make demands on your entire brain and physical system; and at levels of high desire and stress, the game forces on you extraordinary self-integration and self-discipline. Becoming sharp at table tennis is one excellent way to "turn on" more of your midbrain. Other physically demanding, fast-reaction games, such as tennis and the marvelously three-dimensional games of paddle ball and handball, as well as basketball, also are good for your midbrain.

Your midbrain takes the general commands and decisions of your cortex and breaks these down into millions of more specific commands to separate muscles. Imagine how many muscles must be separately commanded, recommanded, and guided in just the right patterned sequence just to carry out your cortical decision to wear a coat. You think nothing of putting on a coat because it requires no thought and *should* require no thought: your midbrain does it for you. Your midbrain moves your myriad muscles of lips, tongue, vocal cords, and chest, so you can think about what you are saying rather than how to shape the sounds to say it. Millions of other tasks you don't usually think about are routinely carried out by your midbrain. You must have a well-functioning midbrain for your cortex to be free to carry out its functions well.

Can you imagine the President of the United States writing every memo and letter, licking every envelope, performing every act now performed by eight million federal employees in thousands of federal agencies? Take away his functionaries and the President could not function as the President. Without your midbrain's working, your cortex could not function either. Improve the way his functionaries work and you will have a better, more effective President. Improve the way your midbrain works and you will have a better, more effective cortex.

In these past few chapters we have talked mainly about the world of sense impressions and movement and physical coordination. But we have talked little about ideas, calculations, and most of the intellectual functions usually regarded as those that make up intelligence. This chapter, too, and parts of several others to come will pay attention to your physical nervous system rather than to the intellectual processes which take place within that system. Like a bad tube, transistor, or circuit connection in your stereo or TV, deficiencies in your nervous system (such as we all have in profusion) sharply reduce the fidelity, range, sensitivity, power, complexity, and general functioning of your intellect. Put the basic equipment into good shape, and development of the intellect can come almost by itself—though, as we shall see, we can do much to spur that intellect development.

So, back to completing more of that task of both-eyes/hand coordination that you began as an infant and later discontinued.

At the top and bottom edges of our field of vision we can follow right or left hand from both eyes. With finger-counting and manipulative tasks such as described in the first of our chapters on treating the pons, we can carry through ranges of hand-eye coordinative development which we hardly touched on as infants, adding greatly to our brain development. Once activated, a brain circuit or brain cell can and will serve many other functions besides the one which called it into development. The more brain that can be called into play on some situation, the more intelligently the owner of that brain can perform in that situation.

Besides edge-of-vision brain development and besides fast-reaction, total-system-involving complexes such as the game of table tennis or ping-pong, to some extent you can add to the fine detail of your main brain regions for hand-eye coordination. Why should we add fine detail in this or any other areas of brain control and perception? Which is easier to write messages in: a bed of very fine sand or a bed of coarse gravel? To the extent that we add to the brain's capacity for handling things in fine detail, we extend notably the range, content, quantity, quality, subtlety, depth, value, and import of the information which that brain can handle.

So, to refine both-eyes/hand coordination: Perform finer and finer tasks of manipulation with each hand in turn, comfortably within the field of vision of both eyes. (And, to refine your sense of position, perform again what you can of those same manipulative tasks, but with your eyes shut.) Unraveling fabrics, threading smaller and smaller needles fixed in a clothespin or clamp of some sort, throwing or shooting darts at a target, erecting houses of playing cards—these and many other suitable single-hand activities come readily to mind.

Then, as before, perform these and other such tasks using *both* hands together in the field of vision. You probably won't gain very markedly in dexterity (after all, you already did a lot of this sort of manipulation as a young child), but any gains you do make in refinement, even barely detectable gains, are important to the information-handling capacity and fidelity of your brain. But you should make at least a little gain in dexterity by doing these things, if only because you are doing them while you are doing so many other things to your brain during your three-week marathon. Your work in dexterity aids both midbrain and cortex.[2]

Using a Boy Scout's manual or other source as a guide, use both hands together in learning a variety of knots to tie and untie, in rope, string, and fine thread, and practice each until it becomes easy for you.

---

2. Together with vision, dexterity is one of the best indicators of the physical condition of your brain. If you find you have *lost* a lot of dexterity since infancy, check immediately with your physician for the possibility of a brain tumor, and for the possibility of the midbrain disorder known as athetosis (until recently thought incurable and progressive, athetosis is now routinely cured at Philadelphia's Institutes for the Achievement of Human Potential)—the earlier such things are caught, the better. If you find merely poor dexterity with no loss from childhood, then these exercises will help you to clear away an important bottleneck in your brain's development.

Thread finer and finer needles, this time using both hands, by holding the needle in one hand instead of a clamp.

To enlist the aid of visual interest, acquire or borrow some highly attractive gemstone. Hold it up and slowly turn it to admire the play of light, at all points of your field of vision and at all distances within and up to arm's length, for a few minutes each day. Experiment with lining it up with other features of visual interest and with crossing beams from several pencil flashlights. Also, experiment with looking through the gemstone at different things—including the reflection of the gemstone in a mirror.

String games, such as cat's cradle, are also good two-hand/both-eye practice and can be found described in books in every public library.

The work you did in fashioning cutouts for your side-vision and general pons development also is good exercise for this coordinative function of your brain.

Tracking moving objects can also stand some practice. Suspend a pencil flashlight with two strings, front and back, from an overhead fastening, to swing back and forth—at first on long strings for longer, slower arcs, later on hitched short for faster pendulum tracking. In the dark, follow the strings right and left, away from and near you. Better still, if you have a partner, have him move the flash up and down, across, around, and in front of you at various distances. Let him bring the flash from some distance away up to your nose and back many times with your eyes fastened on it. Have him vary speed, direction, pattern, distance.

Similarly, holding the flashlight yourself, work the same exercises on yourself as just described for a partner. Why both? "Passive pursuit," where the visual target is moved around for you, and "active pursuit," where you move your target around for yourself, involve different areas of the brain and both should be practiced and improved.

The listening and touch exercises described in the previous chapters benefit midbrain and cortex as well as pons.

It was with your third, reptile-up-on-all-fours brain, your midbrain, that you began as an infant to discover the third dimension—the vertical. It was with your midbrain that you began using both eyes focused together to see in stereo depth.

Of all of nature's programs for developing hand-eye coordination and stereo vision coordinated at arm's length, the most important one by far is hands-and-knees creeping, as noted earlier in this book.

Adult though it be, your brain isn't all that settled down and hard to change. Even before your effort to boost your brain's abilities, you were open to impressions, able to learn things—each such experience made physical changes in your brain, within certain bounds. Now, with everything slammed into this three-week marathon, those bounds have receded. Your brain's resistance to change is temporarily used up, and it is almost as malleable as the brain of a growing infant. Seize the moment and creep, creep, creep! Two tough hours of creeping each day throughout those three weeks!

Obviously, creeping is a pattern of motor actions and sensory feedbacks which involves much more of the brain than just hand-eye, though the hand-eye link may be the most important aspect. At first it may be necessary to hold your attention away from how you are creeping (as you did at first with stomach-to-floor crawling), and simply *move* forward on hands and knees any old way, just to let the pattern and rhythm build itself up and become comfortable. Once your creeping pattern becomes well established and comfortable (and this may take a day or two), switch your attention to it. Soak in the look and feel and even the sound of creeping, soak in the feel of the floor and of movement and slide of skin, muscle, hands, shoulders, arms, belly, toes, haunches, and your head's position relative to both body and floor—feel/see/hear all these things as distinctly as possible, then try to merge them into a single, whole unit of consciousness moving about the floor, with no element left out of the one integrated awareness.

Arrange as extensive and varied a creeping-course as possible: different kinds of floor surface to cross, chairs, tables, and other objects to loom three-dimensionally in your approach and to slide past as you continue your course.

To give variety after the first few days, use tape, pins, or other markers to lay out various courses and tracks to maneuver around and through. In your second and third weeks you may experiment with the pace, speed, and manner of your creeping, but during your first week let the basic pattern become fully established. Another good idea is to heighten hand-eye interest from time to time with different-colored gloves, rings, or even cigar bands, or other hand decorations for your eyes to light upon.

Wear old jeans for your creeping, lay in a good stock of slap-on or iron-on patches for the knees, which will wear through about every other day. Lay in several sets of Ace bandages and wear one around each knee, under your jeans, until your knees toughen. These Ace bandages too will wear through, but not so quickly as the pantsleg.

Two hours of this creeping a day? He's got to be kidding! But this creeping is essential. At the end of the three weeks you will still have gotten in only a total of forty-two hours of creeping, where the healthy and unrestricted infant, with his growing and impressionable brain, will get in dozens of times more creeping on his way to becoming a civilization-builder. We would say creep four hours a day, even six, but this would take too much time away from your other brain-building activities which are also necessary—and because you simply aren't as strong in this respect as is a little baby, your physique probably could not stand up (at first) to a six-hour-a-day creeping regimen. In time you could toughen up enough to keep up and even surpass that little baby, but time is one thing that is all too scarce during this three-week marathon.

Why compress all this activity into three weeks? Why not stretch it out over a longer period of time so it won't be so wearing?

1) Your brain is adult, "settled down," resistant to change. But it can put up only so much resistance to change. If you throw at your brain less concentrated stimulus than it can resist, your brain will stay largely unchanged. Once you give it more than it can resist, you can change your brain readily. It takes almost as concentrated a regimen to change your brain a little as to change it a lot. Spacing out your efforts

into an easier schedule would almost completely waste those efforts.

2) Fortunately for you, the first few weeks of any such brain-building activity are the most productive. Except for delayed-action effects (such as newly trained side-vision areas of the brain gradually and cumulatively beginning to participate in the activities of the main-line centers), most of the effects of your brain-building will come at or near the beginning of the time you override your brain's resistance to change. By the end of three weeks, you will have accomplished a full one third to one half as much as you could if you kept up this extraordinary marathon for an entire year. (Another three weeks would accomplish another full fifth or quarter.)

3) You can maintain almost anything for three short weeks, even as difficult a regimen as this brain-building marathon. If you want to go on for longer, fine: we applaud you, and you will benefit from doing so. But aiming for longer and finding, early in your marathon, that you simply can't keep this sort of thing up for six to eight weeks makes you too likely to abandon the marathon after only a few days and before much is accomplished. Three weeks is realistic and within clear reach. Aim squarely for those three weeks, no more, no less. If, at the *end* of those three weeks, you feel like going on awhile, that is a different matter. Three weeks are also manageable from the standpoint of most vacation schedules.

However forgotten it may be to us now, growing up was hard work. Increasing brain power, as the side-vision exercises, crawling, and creeping will have convinced you by now, is very tough work for you, the adult, quite possibly among the toughest tasks you have performed in your life. Some of it is easy, but some, one may now appreciate, is hard, and keeping up the whole thing for three weeks is also hard work. Make no doubt about it: this marathon is a real test of character (which in the long run counts as much as, if not more than, intelligence).

Aside from creeping, the most noteworthy function of your midbrain, which thrusts your experience into the vertical (third) dimension, is that of balance. The ordinary apartment or household lacks most resources for development of this sense, so your neighborhood or community gym is the place to turn for much of this. Even so, there are things you can do in your home which are suited for lower regions of your cortex and which we will discuss in the next chapter. At the pool in your gym you can do many things in your underwater swimming to stretch and develop your sense of orientation and balance—swimming around and around in a vertical circle, for example, or maintaining yourself upside down. In shallower water you can practice handstands. Learning to dive, and learning various dives, are excellent for developing your sense of orientation and balance.

In the gym itself, possibilities are almost unlimited. There your general rule is this: hang upside down from anything you can, for as long as you can, and maneuver upside down on it for as long as you can. If any bystander becomes curious, explain that you are treating a vestibular problem (vestibular lobes of the cerebellum control the sense of balance)—he won't know what you mean, but he'll think you have explained it, as in a sense you have. If he presses you, tell him that it's something related to the inner ear (which is the sense organ from which the vestibular lobes derive their information about your position). Since that bystander no doubt thinks he knows what the inner ear is and does, this should almost certainly satisfy him. It is not very advisable to let on around the gym crowd that you are engaged in raising your intelligence. They probably still have the shyness and doubts that you once had and would offer at least a verbal resistance.

In that gym or elsewhere, hanging upside down on a single suspended rope, swinging and twirling, will be especially demanding on your brain circuits. It will help them to develop, especially if you swing toward and away from and past some specific visual target on which you can stay oriented. Also, from time to time swing upside down with your eyes closed, soaking in every impression you can from all your other senses. A total of a half to three quarters of an hour a day spent upside down, and doing things while you are upside down, is recommended.

Another advantage of your upside-down activity, besides building neglected areas of the balancing centers in your brain, is the resulting improvement in circulation throughout your entire brain, bringing countless cells and circuits better nutrition, food energy, and oxygen supply.

More demanding activities, such as forward and backward rolls, jumping rope, cartwheels, and headstands, are okay if you can do them or if a bystander or an instructor will help you. Learning the parallel bars or other such gym equipment is more demanding still, and probably beyond the scope of your three-week marathon, unless you already happen to have some experience and skills in those activities.

Caution, and a very important one: If you are elderly, or have ever had a stroke, check very carefully with your physician before undertaking *any* upside-down and/or gymnastic exercise. True, many yogis in their eighties and nineties practice hours-long headstands, but this writer suspects that they began those activities as much younger men and remained accustomed to it.

Your sense of balance involves a most strange area of your brain and midbrain—your cerebellum, which consists of huge brain lobes at the back of your head. The cerebellum dominates the brains of flying birds—who need especially fine balance—as much as the cortex dominates the brains of humans, and may be even more efficient. Brain cells in the cerebellum have one talent that no other brain cells have—magnetic coil induction. In the rest of the brain, one brain cell can affect others or be affected by others only by specific links called synapses. Cerebellar cells not only relate through synaptic links but also wrap around other, unlinked cells in coils so that the surge of electric current in one cell's firing affects by magnetic induction the electric state of other cells around which it is coiled. This magnetic induction ability adds another full dimension to the complexity of the brain's capabilities, to the point where one would almost suspect that, in the long run, birds' superdevelopment of the cerebellum lies closer to the truest, most viable path of evolution than does humans' superdevelopment of the cortex. In any event, we too have fairly powerful cerebellums and can, by exercising the sense of balance, further develop, to some extent, those cerebellums.

Your sense of touch is still important at midbrain level, and in addition to identifying household objects in the dark, you can experiment with placing diverse objects in a box or bag and identifying them by feel. Use a wide variety of objects but the more closely similar the objects you can tell apart, the better. For future reference, sometime you might even learn to read Braille, though time can't be spared for much of that in your first three-week marathon. If you can identify by touch what coins you have in your pocket, your sense of touch is pretty good. If you can tell heads from tails on those coins by touch, you're even better. If you can read the dates on those coins by touch, your sense of feel is excellent.

Each higher level in the upside-down pyramid of your brain has added another dimension to your existence and experience. As with the fish, when you were a newborn infant with only cord and medulla—Brain One—functioning, you experienced and lived in only one dimension. You experienced a single point of awareness, upon which impressions impinged, went away, impinged again. This alternation eventually taught you a second dimension—extent—as your pons learned to see outlines and moved you around flat on the floor in a single plane of existence. In the ideal course of brain development, a development whose actual imperfections you are now trying to repair and enrich, after some experience living in a plane, your third brain—the midbrain—got you up on all fours and started you living and experiencing and moving and balancing in three-dimensional space. (See the following chart.)

In the next chapter we will discuss your fourth brain, the cortex, that uniquely human cortex which, in comparison with that of other land animals, is a biological freak (though sea mammals, particularly whales and dolphins, have comparable cortices—and powerful cerebellums as well). With the cortex, we complete sensori-motor development and enter the realm of actual intellect—a fourth dimension, contrasted to the one-dimensional life of your first brain, the medulla, the two-dimensional life of your second brain, the pons, and the vertical, stereo third dimension of experience encountered with your third brain, the midbrain.

Brain part	Brain level	Description of experience
Cortex	BRAIN FOUR	Four dimensions: human has sense of time; retains and uses awareness of things which are not immediately present in his senses.
Midbrain	BRAIN THREE	Three dimensions: reptile or infant sees in stereo, acquires verticality. Objects are solids.
Pons	BRAIN TWO	Two dimensions: amphibian or infant aware of objects with extent across vision. Lives and moves in a plane.
Medulla/Cord	BRAIN ONE	One dimension: impressions impinging on point of awareness in fish or infant.

10
Into Four Dimensions: Your Fourth Brain, the Cortex

The world abounds with popular methods for raising the performance of your fourth brain, the cerebral cortex. Most of these methods—cultural enrichment, dictionary and crossword use, puzzles, logic games, study techniques, etc.—are fairly useful, even though conventional, *if* you have improved your first three brains—medulla, pons, and midbrain—and thereby removed the main bottlenecks constricting the development of your cortex.

Ninety percent of your brain cells are in your cortex—nine billion of them, more or less. Cortical cells are more able to interconnect in greater, complex networks than are any other brain cells, though they lack the midbrain cerebellum's ability to induce current in cells by magnetic coil induction. Researchers have counted thirty thousand synaptic links between one cortical cell and its fellow cells, and many times more than that are obviously possible.

Cortical cells even look different from other brain cells—they wear a much darker insulating sheath than do lower-brain and nerve cells, which wear white coats of fatty myelin, so that the cortex is the "gray matter" in the otherwise white brain.

With all their ability to form complex interconnected networks, the play of the cortex becomes almost like a free-floating energy field and appears capable of almost anything, whereas pathways in lower levels of the brain are more specific and more fixed by biological heritage. Your first, second, and third brains had to learn *particular kinds* of sensori-motor information to function well. In contrast, almost any kind of information can reach the cortex and involve or develop, to some extent, intricate pathways in that cortex, each involving millions of complexly interlinked brain cells. Even so, some specific areas of the cortex need specific kinds of information to function well. Though with the cortex we leap into far wider realms of information stimulus than the sensori-motor, still at some levels of the cortex some biologically important, specific forms of sensori-motor information are needed to let those levels, and the cortex in general, function well.

It is with your cortex that you think, talk, figure problems, appreciate beauty, walk, climb, learn new skills, and even read this page.

Your cortex takes you into the realm of the fourth dimension—time—for now you remain aware of and even act on things which your senses do not presently perceive. You are still aware of what the boss wants next week, what your professor or teacher said would bring a good grade, what your best friend likes about you, what pleases your spouse or next Saturday's heavy date, the deplorable state of the economy, where it's dangerous to cross the street, how doing A *might,* just might, produce B, that the weatherman said showers this afternoon, that your fellow man has walked on the moon.

No other animal is aware of these things, no other animal but man *can* be aware of these things (until we learn new and more powerful ways to stimulate brain growth). That biological freak perched atop the upside-down pyramid of our brain, the cortex, is what makes us human. All other animals live in one, two, or three dimensions: only man lives in four or more, and it is through the cortex that we do so.

It is not our bodies which give us our advantage and added dimension of life, though upright stance, opposable thumb, and highly sensitive hands help. Some animals are bigger and stronger, some are a lot faster on foot or wing, some are smaller but hardier than the human being. Some animals have better eyes than does man. Many are more active. We share the same lower brains with those other animals. But man is the animal with the freak cortex. With that cortex, man is the time-binder; he not only lives in the present but has bound up and carried along the experiences of the past—he is the only animal that can live in the past. He can project his experiences in predictive patterns: man is the only animal that can live in the future.

Our uniquely human, superdeveloped cortex is our organ of awareness for living in the fourth dimension, time.

This fourth brain of ours is *us*. If somebody invented a cortex transplant, would it actually be a cortex transplant or would it be a body transplant? Who would go home with whose wife? For the most part, my cortex is *me*.

When someone purports to measure your intelligence, what he is measuring is, mainly, the responses of your cortex. These responses determine nearly all of what you do in your schooling, on the job, or with your friends.

Your cortex can work well or poorly, and many things affect how it works. The end purpose of all that you have done to expand the abilities of your lower brains is to improve the functioning of your cortex.

Some of your exercises, especially in touch, smell, position, and hearing, have already aided your cortex directly, as well as indirectly by improving your lower brains. In particular, the more adept you can become at telling apart and identifying closely similar objects in all your senses, the more you are improving the information-handling abilities of your cortex.

Below that level of four-dimensional awareness, there are still more sensori-motor improvements to make in your cortex. The average household has in it one common device which makes especially easy some cortical improvements in stereo vision and in hand-eye coordination: the phonograph turntable. If you don't have a phonograph turntable, borrow one, get an old, second-hand one cheap, or buy a child's portable phonograph for just a few dollars.

Fashion a few dozen roughly circular, foot-wide white discs from cardboard, with a hole in the middle and some sort of weight to fit over the centerpiece in the turntable to hold the disc down against the turntable. Small weights fastened around the lower edge of each disc are an acceptable alternative.

With a magic marker, trace an inch-wide circle near the outer rim of the cardboard disc. Now start the turntable and disc rotating. With the same or a different-colored magic marker, try holding the marker in the center of the smaller circle as it goes around. Visual feedback in the form of stains from the marker pen will quickly tell you how well you are doing, and will underscore that message once you've stopped the turntable a minute later. Draw another inch-wide circle in an as-yet relatively unmarked part of the disc, and try again. When your cardboard disc becomes too marked up by your tracking magic marker to be of further use, flip it and start over. When it's used up on both sides, put it aside and start another disc. About five one-minute trials with your writing hand, three times a day, and three one-minute trials with your nonwriting hand, three times a day, should provide some excellent development in your cortex. (If you run more such trials a day, keep a two-to-one ratio in favor of the hand you write with.)

If you can change the speed on your turntable from time to time, so much the better.

Practice reading labels on your records as they turn on your turntable, for perhaps five minutes a day. If these labels prove too difficult for you, attach larger, more easily read labels to some of your used-up cardboard discs and practice reading them as they turn—and see if before the three weeks are up you can't also read rotating record labels.

Place that turntable so that you can comfortably place your eyes level with it and sight across it at variously spaced objects in the room, and through an open doorway or window at some much more distant scene. On one of your used cardboard discs, cement a half dozen one- or two-inch-tall figurines or objects on various parts of the disc ranged from the center to the edge. With your nose almost against the turntable, rotate the disc and visually track each of the figures on it.

Frequently sight beyond at other, more distant objects in the room and back to the figures, and sometimes sight beyond all this through to the open doorway or window at the more distant scene and back. After the first day or so, swing some highly visual object on a string back and forth in your field of vision a few feet beyond the turntable; look at that and back to the figurines on the rotating turntable frequently. Later in the three-week marathon, add a second pendulum object, and later still a third, at different distances, with different angles and periods of swing.

This near and far ranging and tracking, as you can well imagine and will soon experience, places extraordinary demands upon your cortex and should do much to improve its development. Three fifteen-minute sessions a day are recommended, and a different one at night as follows:

Cement bright-colored figurines on a blackened disc. Focus a lamp on the turntable top so that very little light escapes elsewhere. As described in the previous chapter, suspend a pencil flashlight by strings front and back to swing a few feet away. Arrange a backdrop of flashing Christmas-tree lights at various distances. Keep the rest of the room dark. With figurine disc rotating under the focused light, pencil flashlight swinging, and the Christmas-tree lights flashing, sight on and track every lit visual object in turn in rapid succession, repeating for fifteen minutes.

To involve more of your cortex in the identification and tracking, give each figurine a name and memorize that name, then identify that figurine each time your eye turns to track it.

After a few days of these turntable exercises, you will hardly be able to help noticing that you see everything around you much more quickly and in finer detail. Continue these exercises for the three weeks, but not for very much longer, though, as the limited motions of your phonograph turntable would soon stop aiding your development. If you can invent *other* visual coordinative exercises for tracking in different patterns and directions, then continuing in some form would be worthwhile.

There is a most invaluable thing you can do with your sense

of hearing if you have, or can obtain, the right equipment: a fairly good microphone, a sound amplifier of some sort whether in a component sound system, record player, tape recorder, or cassette, and a good set of headphones.

Rig this equipment so that when you speak into the microphone the sound is carried to the amplifier and comes directly and clearly to the headphones. With headphones on, talk or read into the microphone for fifteen minutes to one hour each day. You will also want to repeat this exercise just before chatting with friends or making a sales pitch or a recitation of some sort, even outside of your three-week brain-building marathon. Here is why:

Electronic feedback—from your voice to the microphone to the amplifier to the headphones to your ears—is much faster than ordinary auditory feedback through the air and through convection within your head. You will find that with faster feedback, your speaking and thinking both clarify and come faster and easier. (By contrast, with tape-loop delay in your feedback, like talking in an echo chamber or in a hall with miserably poor acoustics, your speech and thoughts would become hopelessly muddled.) Speak long enough with electronic-speed feedback, and the clearing and speeding of both your talking and thinking will last for a while afterward. Use this electronic-speed feedback long enough and often enough, in conjunction with your other brain-building activities during your marathon, and your talking and thinking will likely be permanently improved to a noticeable degree.

Jogging is useful to your cortex in two ways. First, it places oxygen-supply demands on your total system and temporarily raises your CO_2 levels (opening the valves in the carotid arteries feeding your whole brain), thereby helping your whole system to better supply your brain.

Second, running and walking are important centers and networks in your cortex which involve and develop much of your brain. To develop these centers further aids your cortex. You probably practice enough walking in your daily activity, except for one special form we will discuss shortly. But chances are that you don't get enough experience running, so that daily jogging will add significantly to the sensori-motor experience and underlying structural integration of your cortex.

Doing a lot of running will improve the pattern of your running and, more important, will improve the efficiency and effectiveness of that vast sea of interlinked cortical circuits involved in walking and running.

Most books on jogging advise you to run not so fast as you can in a sprint but at a lope slow enough for you to sustain the pace for a fair distance. A half-mile jog each day the first week, a mile jog each day the second week, and a two-mile jog each day your third week is probably well within your ability. Needless to say, such jogging will make you look and feel a lot better and improve your physical health, entirely aside from all the mental benefits.

If you walk fairly crisply, gracefully, or smoothly, then the jogging should take care of most of what your cortex still needs in its walking and running centers. If you do not have such a walk, chances are that the jogging will soon give you that desirable walk. If by the end of the first week you still walk poorly, an exaggerated version of the normal walk may be in order.

The normal walk is a motion called "cross-pattern," where left arm swings forward when the right foot does, and right arm swings forward with the left foot. Practicing an exaggerated form of this cross pattern for a half hour a day should erase the imperfections from your walk and improve your cortex.[1] Actually point the index finger of your left hand at your right foot as it comes forward, then the index finger of your right hand at your left foot in turn, and look at where you are pointing. This should correct and enrich the cortical patterns which control your walking, and make your cortex generally more efficient.

---

1. Walking being an activity of the cortex, you can use your cortex —deliberate, conscious attention and contrivance, following closely detailed instructions if necessary—to change or improve your walking-running patterns. Such conscious attention will aid cortical patterns, where it would have crippled the forming of suitable patterns in lower levels of the brain.

Another motor activity extremely important to the cortex is one you may have missed entirely, and certainly one that the usual living patterns do not feature much: climbing and handhold-swinging or brachiation.

Brachiation—hanging suspended and swinging from overhead handhold to overhead handhold—involves a shockingly large portion of the cortex, with complex circuits involving intimately every sense and many kinds of awareness, peripheral awarenesses, and coordination.[2] If you did not get much brachiation as a child, then to practice it now is no less than crucial to further development of your cortex!

Gym facilities are usually available; if not, suspend an old ladder between two uprights.[3] If no ladder is available, a pole or even a pipe will work well. Wear gloves at first until your hands become used to brachiation. If your hands and arms aren't strong enough at first to support your own weight, rig your handholds near enough to the ground or floor for you to get a little support from your tiptoes; gradually raise one end of that set of handholds. Watch your hands as you dangle your way from handhold to handhold. Forty to sixty minutes a day of brachiation in short practice sessions, and another ten to twenty minutes a day of simply hanging by your hands, should greatly aid your cortex, and your chest, respira-

---

2. It is understandable, though, that brachiation should involve such extraordinarily vast areas of the brain, in view of the range of things our tree-swinging ancestors had to keep aware of as they swung from tree to tree over many millions of years. If those ancestors did not notice the hidden weakness of that branch they were reaching for, or did not gauge the distance correctly and all the details of their own strength and leap and coordinated hand-grip in relation to that distance, or notice the snake hidden behind the foliage, or notice the smaller branch marginally in the way—if our tree-swinging ancestors did not keep aware of all these and other things in conjunction with their brachiation, they would not have survived to become our ancestors: they would have fallen out of the gene pool onto the jungle floor below.

3. You can even construct a specially suited brachiation ladder from plans obtainable from Philadelphia's Institutes for the Achievement of Human Potential.

tion, and posture as well. The same handholds will do, in many cases, for you to hook your knees over and get in some more valuable experience hanging upside down.

It is hard to believe that this brachiation can mean as much to your brain as it does. Yet brachiation, involving vast complexes throughout the cortex, was for many millions of years the main method by which our ancestors moved around. Our ancestors brachiated so much for so long that it drastically changed the shape of our physical bodies; but brachiating left a far greater impression on our brains. Brachiation is a vast ocean of experiences that human brains simply must undergo if they are to develop any reasonable portion of their potential for seeing, thinking, feeling, being aware.

And brachiation is something which, in our present culture, we just don't usually get much experience in, and so our cortex is badly stunted. A lot of brachiation will boost your intelligence markedly and fill in crucial gaps, about as much as can anything else described in this book. If schools were to include a vigorous regimen of brachiation in their physical-education programs, they might very well drastically reduce their reading problems and their need for remedial special education classes. (If those schools also included a lot of hands-and-knees games for creeping, and a lot of hold-your-breath-under-water swimming, they would suddenly find themselves almost wholly without reading problems, and their appropriations requirements for remedial education would suddenly drop almost to zero—paying, perhaps, for installation of said swimming pool!)

Reading or no, brachiation involves and "turns on" more of your cortex than does any other activity. Next to brachiation, walking-running is probably the best, but you have fewer gaps to fill in here, making much less difference to your brain. More walking and running *do* help your cortex some, but can hardly be compared to the vast effects wrought throughout your cortex by supplying the heretofore missing experience of brachiation. Next to brachiation and walking-running, for involving much of the cortex, is language—hearing, talking, reading, and thinking in language.

Without language to describe what we perceive, we don't

perceive, notice, or think much at all. Two beautiful experiments by Russian psychologist Lev Vygotsky serve to demonstrate this point:[4]

Separating two groups of very young children according to whether their vocabularies contained words for color, Vygotsky played with them a "shell game" involving two green caps, one red cap, and a piece of candy hidden under the red cap. Children who had color words in their vocabulary followed the game with boring ease. Children without words for colors simply could not follow the red cap in that shell game. In another context Vygotsky taught the latter group of children words for color and then, sometime later, played the shell game with them again—this time that once-failed group also followed the red cap with boring ease.

In another classic experiment, Vygotsky separated children on the basis of whether they had in their vocabularies the words *triangle, dot, slash,* and the like. Then he set both groups to the task of drawing butterfly wings. The children who had word-names for the features characterizing those butterfly wings drew those wings well, could even draw them from memory. The children who had no words for those features flopped hopelessly. Once they learned those words, those hitherto failing children were as successful as the first group, even drawing well from memory what they previously could not draw even while looking directly and closely at what they were trying to draw. Having words for what they were looking at enabled them to *see* what they were looking at.

Without a language, of course, we could not live in the fourth dimension, we could not "bind time:" we could not bundle up our experiences and carry them along, or pass them on to succeeding generations in a cumulating snowball of cultural heritage. But language does help us perceive, as Vygotsky's experiments have shown.

If we have a word for some subtle aspect of existence, or

---

4. Vygotsky, Lev, *Thought and Language* (Cambridge, Massachusetts: The M.I.T. Press, 1962). Translation of a Russian book published in the 1920s, another decades-long delay the advance of science can ill afford.

even a hypothetical, imaginary aspect, we can fix our attention as fully upon that hidden but possibly crucial aspect as upon a louder aspect demanding more attention from our senses.

And how many aspects of even a doorknob can be usefully described, depending on the situation? A thousand? A million? Two million? We *can* distinguish, on the average, seven million different colors (though we have only a few dozen color names in our vocabularies). How could we possibly live in a culture and society, much less contribute to it, if we did not have words with which to bring before our attention myriad subtle aspects of the things with which we have to deal?

On the whole, the bigger our working vocabulary, the more things and aspects we can perceive, and the more intelligently we can function (we'll talk more about that question in the next chapter). Other factors enter in as well, of course: the wealth or paucity of visualized experience associated with each word; whether the concepts, objects, relationships, and classifications named are the most useful to what we need to perceive; and other such matters which we will take up soon.

Again, those aspects of language in which we already have plenty of experience and practice—talking and hearing—can hardly be improved, but even there we have seen that electronically speeded feedbacks using microphone, amplifier, and headphones can make a significant difference in our thinking ability. Reading is the aspect of language experience we are least likely to get enough of, and so in the next chapter we will discuss it.

It is not just the content of information in your brain, but how well it is organized, that makes a big difference in how well you function. It is one thing to have a well-sorted filing cabinet, another thing altogether to have all the papers in that cabinet jumbled in a heap.

The human cortex, in contrast to the brains of other animals, has had to handle so much information that a few hundred thousand years ago it invented a filing system we call "cerebral dominance." Our brains are divided into two halves front-to-back, a left and a right pair of hemispheres (oddly, perhaps for mechanical strength within the brain structures themselves, the right hemisphere controls the left side of the body and the left hemisphere the right side).

If a person is right-handed and right-footed and right-eared and right-eyed, or if he is left-handed and left-footed and left-eared and left-eyed, he has successfully established complete cerebral dominance of one brain hemisphere over the other. When we have complete cerebral dominance, the dominant side of the brain controls the hand you write with and stores and handles words, word-concepts, and formal, logical thinking. The other, subdominant side of the brain stores and handles experiences related to the sense of beauty and rhythm, and may be closely involved with intuitive insights. Most sensori-motor decisions, in a well-organized brain, are automatically premade for you, so your attention can go on to other things; you don't have to spend "cortical air time," so to speak, deciding which foot to pull your pants over first, which hand to eat with, which foot to start up the stairs with.

If your brain is *not* well organized, a sort of tug-of-war can result between the two hemispheres of your brain: "H-h-here, I-I'll t-t-t-take the b-b-ball"—"N-no I-I-I'll t-t-take it!" This can happen if, say, you are right-handed but left-eyed and -footed, or ambidextrous, or otherwise don't have your skills sorted and lined up on the proper side of your body. This condition is called "mixed dominance." Mixed cerebral dominance is the cause of most cases of stuttering, and of many problems in poor coordination, slow and uncertain movement, and accident-proneness. This has been the case so often that you can easily read up on how to identify and correct the condition. Frankly, though, *unless* you stutter or have serious problems in coordination, it would be better to let alone the whole question of cerebral dominance. But lately there has been incidental evidence that in many instances of apparent mixed dominance the brain devises a newer, more sophisticated filing system which is better than the one of left-right word-concept/beauty-concept. In these instances a curious cross-linking between word-logic and beauty-intuition has been suggested, leading to the person concerned being highly creative and a highly talented contributor to civilization, whether as scientist, artist, poet, engineer, or administrator.

This new mixed-dominant, more sophisticated cerebral filing system, if it exists and if the incidental evidence gleaned thus far is not misleading, is so much more powerful than the old straight-dominance one that it may well represent a next step upward in human evolution. In any event, despite the now widely spreading conviction found in current literature and among professionals that mixed dominance is a bad thing and should be straightened out at all costs, *unless* it causes you evident problems in speech and/or coordination, you are probably better off with the mixture than without it. This is an excellent reminder that we *don't* know all the answers—in fact we hardly know any of the right questions yet, particularly with regard to the human brain.

Yet we do have much to go on which is of clear benefit to the brain—and if we fail to use it, how shall we ever arrive at the next set of right questions to ask?

11
Information and Cortex

We have talked about physically changing and improving your brain by putting certain kinds of information into it by means of sight, sound, touch, taste, smell, and kinesthetic position-sense. Before we discuss the kinds of information you are used to thinking of as "information"—the kinds of facts, figures, theories, etc., which are in the experience only of humans, in the higher regions of the freakishly superdeveloped cerebral cortex—let's clarify our understanding about what "information" *is.* Here is some information about information:

What do these things have in common?

Rabbit tracks in snow.

A traffic light.

A nod of the head.

The printing on this page.

Each of those things is a "message"—it tells us something, if we know how to read or decode it. If we don't have the information with which to decode or read it—say, if the printing on this page were in Chinese—neither you nor I could understand. The message would be there, but we couldn't get anything from it.

What sorts of things are messages?

The "V-for-victory" sign.

The layers exposed on a cliff face—at least, these are messages to anyone trained in geology.

The bent twig or disturbed leaf, read by the trained hunter.

A different shade of green in part of a cornfield, to an alert farmer.

Thumbs down.

A pat on the back.

The swirl of a galaxy, or the stripes of color on a spectrograph, as read by one trained in astronomy or astrophysics.

Faint praise.

Lipstick on the collar.

A rapidly falling barometer.

At Rhine Institute in Duke University, researchers thought that they had found some real telepaths, people who could consistently read minds by extrasensory perception and tell which of several cards the researcher was looking at. As it turned out, in those earliest instances the perception was not extrasensory: without knowing it, the supposed telepaths were actually reading "body language"—they could tell which card the researcher was looking at from the *way* he was looking.

Let us turn from such sophisticated examples of message-reading to fundamental aspects. When people who are blind from birth are helped by medical science to get their sight, even if their eyes are then fully workable, it takes such people six weeks or longer even to tell the difference, by sight, between a triangle and a circle. It takes that long to build up the visual information experience needed to achieve that small a visual feat (this could be done much sooner and better if the physicians treating such patients were aware of developments in fields other than but adjacent to their own). It can take a child too long to build up such information, so that his at first rapidly growing brain doesn't grow correctly or have the normal level of abilities if he isn't fed the right kinds of visual information at the right times. If he is fed better-than-average quantities and qualities of information at the right times, his brain will be correspondingly better able to read the "messages" of the world around him.

To see, hear, or make sense of any sensory impression at all is a function of what you *already* know and understand. For example, consider all the kinds of previously stored information you require to make sense of seeing a bulge in hanging curtains and a glimpse of a shoe underneath. And depending on the context, you may "read" all kinds of terribly shrewd and sophisticated information from that one visual message.

General Theorem: Every pattern, every configuration, indeed every event in the universe is a "message," if you can acquire the "decoding" information with which to read it.

Suppose all parents taught their children this awareness, even before they entered school—that every pattern, every configuration, every object, and every event in the universe is a message if they have learned or can learn the "decoding" information with which to read it. Suppose each child could grow up with this kind of awareness and expectancy, seeing everything around him through eyes with this kind of consciousness and understanding.

A psalmist realized something along these lines three thousand years ago:

> The heavens declare the glory of God
> And the firmament shows His handiwork.
> Day after day tells of it,
> Night after night is full of the knowledge.
> There are no words,
> No speech of it is heard,
> Yet their voice goes out through all the world
> And their message to the ends of the world.

Has anyone gotten the message?

How can we "get the message" better?

Let us look again at the development of vision. The newborn infant must experience a certain amount of changes in light value—the only kind of seeing which registers on his brain at the time. He must experience changes between light and dark and various colors before he can begin to notice light-value differences between different areas of what he is looking at—that is, before he can begin to see outlines and profiles. He must experience seeing many changes in light value before he can develop a code which will enable him to decipher more of the visual information available to him—before he can generalize these experiences enough to begin to notice and respond to outlines, a "higher code" of visual information. This higher code permits the same visual act to take in many times more information than was handled before, to extend visual experience and facility by a full order of magnitude over what went before. And yet this higher-coded experience of outline perception could not have emerged without being preceded by a quantity of lower-code information (changes in light value) which was great enough to permit generalizations that coded into the next higher level of experience.

Similarly, that infant needs a vast amount of experience at seeing outlines before he can generalize that information into a code which permits him to see and respond to simultaneous outlines and smaller configurations *within* the larger outlines. In other words, by such code-building experience the visual centers of his brain code at increasingly sophisticated levels, permitting him to see in finer and finer detail, to build perception of minute differences between the detail seen with the right eye and that seen with the left, so that the infant adds yet another dimension and range to his vision by seeing in stereo, and so on.

A simpler example and one closer to experiences you are still aware of: learning to ride a bicycle. Recall, by feel and by memory, how the demanding task of staying upright and in motion became an utterly trivial and insignificant part of the comprehensive, variegated, and generally pleasant range of experience of riding a bicycle, and you will have a better feel for the point we are about to make. If you review, by feel and memory, your similar progression in other skill-demanding tasks such as driving, playing a musical instrument, dancing, public speaking, painting, writing, and so on, you will better understand the point we are about to make. A further example is handwriting: the more fortunate among us learned to read and write at such an early age that they cannot remember what it was like to be unable to read or write. But try this experiment, even if you are one of these: s-c-r-a-w-l out your name on a sheet of paper, going very slowly and laboriously, taking at least a full minute to complete the task. As you finish, pay close attention to the feelings you are experiencing and the early memories this has brought back to you. As you consider the range of difference between your glibly writing a letter today and the time when you had no opportunity to pay attention to phraseology, when you had to give all your effort and attention to making the words and even each letter come out right, the point we are about to express will mean more to you.

The point is this: Experience at any level depends on having a "code" built out of and generalized from the store of experience on the level below it. Each level provides at least a full order of magnitude of experience, competence, control over a vaster range of things than does the level beneath it. Each level can, in turn, through much experience, generalize a code with which to build a next-higher level of experiencing.

We know of no ceiling on this progression.

We know of no such limits, but we do know a drag on this progression, imposed by limits on self-expectation, by what we have observed of other people, and by what other people expect of us.

With the higher levels of the human cortex we ascend from merely sensory and motor information into that vast continuum of purely human areas of consciousness and experience. That continuum ranges upward from the first, fumbling understandings arrived at when, as tots, we were first learning to put together a few words in differing combinations, to the most powerful and sophisticated conceptualizations about self, mankind, lifekind, and the universe that the greatest minds among us have formulated—and beyond.

Some concepts are better than others, regardless of level.

For example, Cro Magnon man was far more intelligent than we, but the caveman concepts he had to work with were not nearly so useful as the concepts we have to work with today. We, physically and mentally inferior to Cro Magnon man, can nevertheless out-think him and accomplish far more on a vastly superior scale—because, after ten thousand years of more or less cumulative civilization, our concepts are better than his.

In line with this argument, within our own culture some areas of conceptualization have recently emerged which can bring us gains similar to those in the comparison between presentday and Cro Magnon cultures. For various reasons these new modes and levels of thinking and perceiving have not yet entered very deeply into the rest of our culture; chances are that you have not even heard of them. Yet Information Theory, such as much of this chapter is based upon, and Cybernetics or General Systems Theory provide a means to generalize all present scientific information and experience into integrated "higher codes" for experiencing and acting upon things, at a higher and more general level of comprehension and effectiveness.

You can gain at least a little effectiveness from these new areas of conceptualization, even if your level of intelligence remains otherwise unchanged, by re-examining the first few pages of this chapter. But combining fresh awareness of these new areas with the gains in intelligence you will otherwise be obtaining from the suggestions in this book should lead to some interesting further gains.

Another, and more specific, way in which the considerations in this chapter affect you:

Present a three- to six-year-old child with two clear glasses, one much larger than the other. Fill the smaller one with water until full. Pour—or have him pour—the contents of the smaller glass into the larger one, which because of its greater volume remains half-empty. Ask the child: "Is the amount of water now greater than, less than, or the same as it was when it was sitting in the other glass?"

Chances are that the child will tell you the water is now

less, because the glass it is now sitting in is partly empty and the other one had been full.

Pour the same water back into the smaller glass, filling it once again, and chances are that the child will tell you that now there is more water, because the glass holding it is full.

No, there is nothing wrong with the child. His answer is wrong, but perfectly in keeping with the concepts he has at this stage of development. Until he encodes from enough experience at pouring quantities back and forth between containers, he will not realize that the amount of water is conserved—that the quantity is the same regardless of the container in which it is held. He will not have encoded the concept of conservation of matter, which in turn will permit him to perceive and relate to a vast range of other phenomena involving constancies.

The point of this? You *can,* by dint of persuasion, adult authority, demonstration, *teach* that child the *fact* that the amount of water remains the same regardless of the container. *If* you succeed in doing so, you will in fact have crippled that child's mind, for he thenceforth can never *see* in that vast range of related phenomena as well as if he had discovered that fact/principle for himself.

The point is this: For too large a proportion of those basic experiences in early key concepts, the American school—the one you and I attended and the one your children go to or will attend—is in the business of *teaching* children the *fact* that the amount of water remains the same regardless of whichever container is holding it!

That, specifically, is the reason why you and I are crippled in our perceptions and conceptualizations. *That,* specifically, is the reason why so few people can see much for themselves and must, instead, depend on other people's opinions.

What can we do about this terrible and inexorable crippling of our minds? Not very much. Elsewhere,[1] this writer has proposed a form of "concept-therapy" or "cognitive therapy"

1. See chapters 4, 6, and 7 of Wenger, Win, *On Raising Human Intelligence* (Federalsburg, Maryland: MCM Press, 1971).

wherein the models of mental development proposed by Jean Piaget and/or Jerome Bruner are made the basis of diagnostic tests to measure the strong and weak areas of the patient's concept-development. To cure the areas of weakness, the therapist would hypnotize and "regress" the patient to the earliest levels of a sector of experience which he was failing to really grasp for himself. In that hypnotically regressed state, and with subjective experience of time greatly expanded by the same hypnosis, the patient would be led to experience afresh and for himself the key principle at issue and to integrate this new, self-held understanding into all his areas of experience subsequently dependent upon it. Theories and some evidence argue persuasively that such cognitive therapy would make dramatically large improvements in the workings of anyone's intelligence—but to date not one professional researcher or therapist other than this writer has shown the slightest flicker of interest in this line of possibilities, and *no* resources have been made available for its development. If suddenly the line of study were fully opened and many people plunged into its work, it would still be some years before the fruits of that labor would become available to you.

Aside from cognitive psychotherapy, subjective time-expansion under hypnosis, especially under self-hypnosis initially and carefully guided by a responsible professional, should add greatly to your effectiveness in other regards as well. As with dreams which seem to last a lifetime but go on for only an instant, subjective time-expansion under hypnosis can gain you hours of inner experience in only a few seconds. With this technique well developed under your control, all you'd need for respite or for figuring out a problem would be to push a mental button and suddenly find you had all the time in the world for coping with the situation, no matter how pressing.[2, 3]

---

2. Cooper, Linn F. and Erickson, Milton H., *Time Distortion in Hypnosis* (Baltimore: Williams & Wilkins, 1954).

3. Masters, Robert and Houston, Jean, *Subjective Realities*. Private monograph, undated but originating *c.* 1972–73.

Since cognitive psychotherapy has been denied to you by the lack of interest prevailing in the profession, what *can* you do about the way your mind has been crippled by the teaching you have received? Mainly, you have two very general recourses:

1) *Visualizing*. Picture to yourself, in as sharp detail as possible, some of the matters before your attention which are presently described in words or formulas. If you are a student, extract key points from the most abstract, abstruse or difficult of the subjects you are now studying and try to fix them as graphically and as closely as possible to the level of personal experience in your consciousness. If you consider the matters in this book to be of some importance, you might wish to visualize and make as graphic as possible some of the theories stated in these pages, including this chapter's "General Theorem," or its thesis, stated subsequently, of coding at different levels of experience.

If you have or can borrow a tape recorder, and obtain from an audio distributor a repeating reel or cartridge with a five- to ten-minute cycle of repetition, you can considerably strengthen this line of effort. Record on the reel a verbal description of the principle perception which you are trying to deepen. Start it playing back; lie back and "blank" your mind for a few cycles—then start paying attention to the principal and begin visualizing what it is that is being described. For some people this procedure works much better when the already-recorded reel is started on its playback immediately upon awakening in the morning.

2) *Reading*. Read a lot of what you *most enjoy* reading. Whether it's sex, comic books, mysteries, travel, pot-boilers of various ilks, or whatever, just go ahead and read a lot of it for a while. Build up toward a day when you "saturate" on that type and level of reading, then take a day's break and (possibly with a librarian's help) locate fresh books in the same field of interest but which are a little more informative, theoretical, and/or challenging than the line you've just saturated in. This procedure should let you code in enough experience in your most-preferred areas to encode comfortably

to a higher level, and to begin winning correspondingly greater reward from your reading. Simply forcing your way through a book not comfortable for you, as so often happens with schooling, does not usually "turn people on" to reading. Instead, saturate in what you enjoy reading. Before that starts to lose spark for you, you should have enough basis to enjoyably and comfortably encode to the next higher—and more rewarding—level.

We cannot emphasize strongly enough that reading is good for you neurologically and in terms of your mind's life. Nearly all the worthwhile experiences, observations, ideas, feelings, and aspirations of the human race have been recorded in print. Reading puts you in communication with humanity's greatest minds. Much of that reading can equip you with a sophistication of language in which to think and perceive—remember those experiments of Lev Vygotsky cited earlier? Truly, reading is fundamental to much of the experience of being human.

If you have found reading tiring, difficult, or hard to sustain, many of the sensori-motor exercises described earlier in this book should improve that. Even during your three-week brain-building marathon, and for a long time thereafter, take advantage of this gain to stock your reopened mind with *comfortable* reading.

If you can work your way up to a regimen of two or three books a day, then settle, for the long haul, into a pattern of at least two or three books a week, you probably have it made.

To your reading, add biographies and autobiographies, either of very intelligent and admirable people or even geniuses, or of people who scored admirable successes in what you are now trying to accomplish. After particularly interesting accounts of the lives of such people, accounts which get inside the person enough to show him as a human being and to detail the circumstances in which he was working (even if, as in some instances, it is a fictional novel or even a fictional character), begin to extend the action in your mind's eye a little further, from some particularly interesting situation, the one which had most seemed to come alive for you out of those described. Fantasize new situations with the same character playing a role in them. Over a few days' time, fantasize that same admirable character playing a part in situations increasingly similar to your own. Then stop for a day or so and build the same cycle with another distinctly different but still admirable character.

Put the newer character into the same situation, similar to your own, that you had put the earlier character into. If in this constructive fantasy his actions are characteristically and distinctly different from those of the first, but both sets of actions are plausible, you are probably ready for the next stage. If not, you may have to experiment at this level for a few more days or weeks before moving on. Even at this first stage of role-fantasizing you may be able to turn the imagined actions of your characters to some immediate advantage in your own study, work, or interpersonal circumstance.

The next stage of role-fantasizing is that of putting your imagined character directly into the problems, desires, or other circumstances confronting you. Either picture them playing out their roles in the projected circumstance or picture yourself asking for, and receiving, their advice as to your best course of action. Dale Carnegie credits his most successful decisions to a fantasy technique wherein he imagined certain of the world's greatest minds sitting at a meeting of his personal board of directors. Whenever he had a difficult problem he would go, in his imagination, to this fantasized board of directors and seek the advice of those greatest minds. The answers he got from such fantasy always seemed to work for him.

Why does such fantasy and role-play work so well? It's a way of getting *around* those blocks and habits of self-limitation we all have. Such self-limitations are so closely intertwined with our sense of identity that it is very hard to lift ourselves past those limits. However, our minds are vastly more capable than what we've become accustomed to in ourselves, and will provide startling revelations when we step temporarily into someone else's *persona* in role play, or can fantasize clearly enough the actions of other characters. So powerful are the effects, and so shrewd and accurate is the information generated by such fantasy, that many persons who have used the technique were utterly convinced that they *were* in actual communication with the mind of the person they were fantasizing; it just didn't seem possible that some of the information they received could have been obtained by anything other than actual communication. The belief that the communication was actual does not make it so. These persons simply underrated their own abilities.

The third stage is incorporating into your own personality the new skills and "borrowed" abilities to cope, underscoring again and again in your own mind that it *is* your own brain, your own mind, which has been supplying you with all those extraordinary answers and information, and that the limits on you, which your imaginary characters slipped past or found did not apply to them, do *not* apply to you either because *you* have, in fact, already slipped by them yourself. These three stages should eventually enable you to move about in the real world, accomplishing your aims *your* own way, as readily as did the characters you role-fantasized.

Both American[4] and Russian[5] experimenters have gone a step further in this role-fantasy direction. Students in an art class developed rapidly into advanced, mature, sophisticated artists but with their *own* style when, under hypnosis, during instruction and practice they believed themselves to be Rembrandt, da Vinci, or some other great artist. Other students made similar gains when imagining these sessions of instruction and practice under hypnotic time-distortion, which enabled them to experience subjectively a year or so of intense and profound "instruction" and "practice" within the space of a few minutes. Such techniques appear readily extendable to other fields, but should be undertaken *only* with a most responsible professional already well practiced in those techniques.

---

4. Houston and Masters, *op. cit.*

5. Chapter 12, "Artificial Reincarnation," in Ostrander, Sheila and Schroeder, Lynn, *Psychic Discoveries Behind the Iron Curtain.* (Englewood Cliffs, New Jersey: Prentice-Hall, 1970).

Without hypnosis, and with fairly ordinary role-play, researchers in Sofia, Bulgaria, have gotten extraordinary effects from a set of techniques called "Suggestopedia" or "Cue-Reinforced Learning."[6] Teachers using the method have students assume a different identity and even a different name for the entire time they are in the class, appropriate to what is being studied. A course in the French language, for example, will have one student in the role of, say, Pierre Montaigne, a shopkeeper; another student a French writer, another a French policeman or civil servant, and so on. Maintaining those roles and identities through the course, students slip past their blocks and make extraordinary gains, which non-Bulgarian observers have seen and attested to,[7] and the method is now being tried out in various other countries, among them Canada.[8]

Though other elements in the Cue-Reinforced Learning method also play a part, the use of such role-play to slip past the limitations which appear so integral to our own sense of identity has played at least a strong part in the rapidity with which students learn by this nonhypnotic but role-playing method. Published reports (mostly in Bulgarian) indicate that foreign languages can be easily and comfortably mastered at a rate of from three hundred to a thousand new words a day without strain or fatigue, even by poor students with "no head for languages." Private information now indicates that in some classes the rate has been boosted to more than eighteen hundred words per day. Other special effects, equally notable, appear directly traceable to other aspects of the Cue-Reinforced

6. Lozanov, Dr. Georgi, *Suggestology* (Sofia, Bulgaria: 1971—in Bulgarian). An English edition is in preparation for publication.

7. See, for example, Bancroft, W. J., "Foreign Language Teaching in Bulgaria," *The Canadian Modern Language Review,* Vol. XXVIII (March 1972) pp. 9–13.

8. As a result of Andrews, A., Bélisle, L., Fancy, R., Lortie, R., and Racle, G., "Report of the Canadian Team on Their Stay at the Institute of Suggestology in Sofia" (To the Bureau of Languages, Canadian Ministry of Education, December 20, 1972). Private manuscript, translated from the French by Mankind Research Unlimited, Inc., Washington, D.C., November 1973.

Learning method,[9] but such results, now being replicated in other countries, still seem to point up the extraordinary power of role-play and fantasized roles in helping us slip past self-limitations we didn't even know existed.

Goal-setting, such as in psychocybernetics,[10] can be used to similar effect. The more distinctly and powerfully you can picture your goal, the more everything around you tends to fall into place and move things toward attainment of that goal.[11] It would be of some help, regardless, to clarify just what it is you want in order to work toward it more efficiently, but some elements of this goal-directed psychocybernetics appear to do much the same things as does role-fantasy projection, helping us slip past our self-limitations. For example, one psychocybernetic technique is to picture oneself, as clearly as possible, carrying through in the successful stages of a forthcoming event or task related to his goal. Over and over again, with as strong a visualization as possible, the person practicing this method pictures himself clinching the sale, making the "A," or whatever, building the conviction that this *will* be the outcome. Often, then, things seem to fall into place, and this *does* become the real outcome.

Some techniques appear to require much effort but have some benefits. Straight vocabulary-building will generally raise I.Q. scores by some 10–20 points. One of the favored methods is simply to start going through a few pages of a pocket-sized dictionary each day, marking off and learning the definition of every word whose meaning you can't immediately and specifically recognize. Sliding an index card down the dictionary page, you can retest yourself on all the words you've

---

9. Wenger, Win, and members of the staff of Mankind Research Unlimited, Inc., "Program to Test Cue-Reinforced Learning." Private paper, 1973.

10. Maltz, Maxwell, MD, *Psychocybernetics* (New York: Simon and Schuster, 1968).

11. A literary description of this principle is presented in Hermann Hesse's *Siddhartha* (New York: New Directions Paperbooks, 1957).

marked off—and place an extra mark beside the one which you didn't quite get on the second go-around . . . and so on. In this manner one can expand his vocabulary to include nearly all of what is contained in a pocket or abridged dictionary, and can run up some respectable I.Q. gains in the process. These I.Q. gains from vocabulary-building may also reflect at least a little gain in actual intelligence, in view of the earlier-cited experiments by Lev Vygotsky on the effects of vocabulary on perceiving and thinking.

After one has a good vocabulary, whether from the abridged-dictionary exercise above or by other means, or from previously acquired knowledge, he should undertake reading a comfortable, relatively simple introduction to philosophy. Bertrand Russell's[12] appears to be a good one to start with and will suggest others, as will your librarian. If, after one, or six, or a dozen such books, you reach the point where you can comfortably follow the arguments and even argue with their authors as to their conclusions, you will probably be in excellent shape to handle almost anything else—you have thus acquired not a stock of information but a *way* of thinking.

Logic games, such as Wff-n-Proof (which the writer found, however, hard to get into), capitalize more specifically on raising one's ability to think logically, and some people have claimed I.Q. gains in association with the use of the games. These gains may very well be real in some instances, for the ability to think logically is certainly necessary, and the games provide a basis of exercise for such specific ability. But unless one's intelligence is fairly well developed in other aspects as well, he will tend to fail to transfer skills developed in one activity to other activities. Without good support from other components of intelligence, besides that of formal logical thinking, skills developed in logic games will not even transfer into exercise of logic in other thinking activities, much less bring broader benefits. Logic is a function specifically of the

12. Russell, Bertrand, *The Problems of Philosophy* (from 1912) (New York: Oxford University reprint, 1972).

dominant, usually left side of the cerebral cortex, and to serve well must be well integrated both with well-developed lower regions of the brain and with the subdominant, intuitive-esthetic side of the cerebral cortex. Blanket claims of a person's being able to raise his I.Q. by activities which only in rare instances aid broader intelligence provide several kinds of armament to those in the professional world who wish to deny and prevent any form of intelligence-raising research or activity.

As exemplified by, among other things, the failure thus far to develop cognitive psychotherapy, mentioned above, professionals' disinterest in or distaste for new lines of inquiry outside their own has built up a considerable backlog of new approaches that have some promise but which nevertheless have not come into general use. Some of those techniques have been picked up by groups outside the establishment and run on their own. Many, perhaps most, of the techniques used by José Silva's Mind Control appear in large part to actually aid mental capabilities to an extent which should be respected—and these techniques can be respected no matter what one thinks of the theories propounded alongside them. (Mind Control centers now exist in most major cities and can be located through most telephone directories.) Another set of largely effective, if somewhat more expensive, techniques can be found with Ron Hubbard's Scientology "church." Particularly "word-clearing" with an "E-meter," wherein uncertainties over word meanings are reflected by variations in the subject's electrical skin conductivity and are thus specific targets for immediate "clearing," appears especially effective. At the very least, word-clearing appears to lend a much greater precision of intellectualization and much greater ease of future learning. By removing the clouding caused by confusions, the technique appears to raise intelligence by the equivalent of many points of I.Q., though the degree of separation between Scientologists and more formally respected circles makes hard, reliable data in this regard somewhat difficult to come by. Scientologists have branches of their "church" in many major cities and can be located, too, through phonebooks. (Scientologists also make a wholly unabashed, refreshing, and, to this writer, commendable appeal to people's desire to help humanity.) Because of high prices, and because some Scientological theories and practices appear to him at least to be rather dubious, this writer does not recommend that the reader utilize the services of Scientologists to raise his intelligence—but I cannot in good conscience recommend against this course of action either—caveat emptor. But at least that one word-clearing technique, and probably others, are effective in raising one's intelligence.

The main point here is that an idea should be considered on its own merits, and not (*ad hominem*) on the basis of how one feels about the "ideasmith." That, at least, is the law in the republic of the sciences, but, unfortunately, that law is mostly observed in the breach.

Dr. Georgi Lozanov, discoverer of Cue-Reinforced Learning, said it well: "Disbelief is merely belief with a minus sign in front of it."[13] Skepticism, essential in all matters of science, is one thing; prejudicial rejection is quite another. We have been living through an era of prejudicial rejection—and you, and we, and all of us, have been paying the price for it.

Because we live in an era of prejudicial rejection, communication of really important new discoveries and approaches is very difficult—many such new contributions have no doubt been snuffed out altogether and lost to us. Many others, unknown to this writer, may be gathering force at this moment despite the odds. Many others are known by this writer to be highly promising but simply have had no opportunity to be tested.

Prejudicial rejection operates in more than just the professional and scientific establishments' rejection of new discoveries from outside their ranks. The same dismissal frequently applies between different specialties within the establishment as well; Lozanov's "belief with a minus sign," which has no more legitimate place in the republic of the sciences than does naïvely positive belief, has come to almost totally dominate the affairs of that republic.

---

13. Lozanov, *op. cit.*

With so much rejection of nearly everything, fairly substantial groups of people have gotten into the habit of accepting what the establishment rejects, until we have disseminating through our culture many kinds of new and esoteric notions, some of which are foolish and a few of which may be dangerous. The failure of our truth-seeking institution, the republic of the sciences, to do its job is resulting in a confusing and perhaps disintegrating world where it may soon require, to survive, considerably higher levels of both wisdom and intelligence than now prevail.

The limited hope is that, through what you accomplish with this book, you can not only attain your own goals but also equip yourself to successfully cope with and sort through the confusions now coming upon us. The greater hope is that the worst of those confusions can be averted and that a generally saner and more intelligent population can begin to carve itself a sounder and more rewarding human way of life.

Of the sectors of this book upon which to put the most weight in your efforts, at least initially concentrate on those early chapters dealing with redeveloping the lower levels of your brain. Those lower levels are your most comprehensive bottleneck; expanding the abilities of your lower brain will then make more effective everything you do with your cortex, including the various possibilities cited in this chapter, and including the things you want to do now—and the things you will want to do in the future. For that is the point: Just as improving your lower brain aids all the other things you can do with your brain, improving your brain *per se* is your essential aid to all else. Man's greatest tool is his brain, and you now have the tools with which to improve that tool.

Here's to better experiencing in the future, and a future better worth experiencing!

Appendix: Self-Evaluation

Moving around, which involves all of your senses, is probably more important to the development and structure of your brain than any other function. Each level of your brain has its own special pattern for your moving around. One way to tell how well each level of your brain is working is to test each pattern of movement.

Medulla. Located in the medulla is the source of the most primitive, earliest, and most infantile mode of locomotion, one that has been forgotten or suppressed in most people—underwater swimming. Newborn babies swim well under water if dunked within the first few hours after emerging from the aquatic world in which they spent their first nine months of life. Frequent practice of underwater swimming would tremendously aid the brain development and physical health of most babies, but this privilege appears to be reserved thus far for subnormal, premature infants who, in some hospitals, are given this treatment of underwater swimming as a means to save their lives and bring their health up toward normal—or average. Presumably it never occurred to anyone in this branch of pediatrics that average is not "normal" and that unhandicapped babies will gain still more intelligence and vitality from the same procedure.

Another way to regard the matter is in terms of man's

evolution—back behind the primates, behind the primitive mammals, behind the reptiles and amphibians, he traces his line of descent back through fishlike creatures who swam in Earth's early, warm oceans. You still carry the chemistry of that primeval ocean around with you in your veins. The only working brain that fish have, or that our early sea-swimming ancestors had, is the medulla—and the only motions the medulla knows are swimming and drifting.

So to test your medulla, make like a fish. In your nearest accessible pool, try yourself out on underwater swimming and drifting. If your wind is too short at first to allow you to stay under for more than a few seconds at a time, practice with a "dead man's float" (floating limply, face forward into the water), popping your head up every few seconds for a breath, until your system adjusts to a longer breathing cycle and until you get a bit better feel for keeping your face under water.

And now score yourself. If you can get around comfortably under water, up and down and laterally (you don't have to swim the length of the pool under water or perform other athletic feats), and find yourself feeling pretty much at home there, give yourself an "A" on this function-level and enter that "A" onto the first of the three self-scoring tables following page 125. Enter that "A" in the lower left-hand corner where the row from the left is labeled "Medulla" and the column from the top is labeled "mobility."

If you can manage under water after a fashion but just can't get comfortable at it for whatever reason, if something is always bothering you or throwing you off, give yourself a "B" on this function-level and enter it on the first of the three tables provided.

If this activity is a very difficult one for you, for whatever reason, give yourself a "T" and score it on that table. This is a special *T*arget area demanding special effort and attention from you. You have a bottleneck in your development in this function-level of your brain that has handicapped you in other areas, including areas you may not have suspected. Remove this disability and you have opened the way for important development through a wide range of brain-functions.

And if you can't manage any underwater swimming at all,

score yourself "R" on the table and *R*evert to the next lower level of functioning—which in this instance is the "dead man's float" mentioned above. Practice that float until you can get completely relaxed and comfortable.

A special word at this point: If there is any function-level at which you are unable to perform, revert to the next lower level for that activity on the table and practice that. You have to build into the experience from *below*. Do *not* take lessons or instructions on *how* to perform functions below cortical level. Cortically directed activities remain based in your cortex, and this is not any help to most of those functions or to your brain's development. Anything you can't do readily and automatically, hit at the next lower level and fumble at the problem activity from time to time. Fumble your way into the problem activity, don't think your way through it—unless you are at a cortical-level activity, in which case it *is* useful to use your cortex and think your way through the activity.

The brain has a certain rhythm for recycling ideas, information, experiences. Thirty-six hours after you have struggled with, say, underwater swimming (or with foreign-language learning, one of the first contexts in which this cycle was observed), your brain will have digested some of this experience and will have reached a peak "readiness" to take on and try to handle more of that same experience. Three days—seventy-two hours—after the initial experience, the brain reaches a far bigger and better peak of "readiness," its best peak. Three days to the hour after you've struggled with a task, whatever the nature of that task, you can expect to score your biggest breakthroughs in that task if you take it up again.

Three days to the hour after an underwater swim session or attempt, if you are again wrestling with that task at that time, you may expect to make your biggest breakthroughs. This is not to say that you should space your trial sessions at three-day intervals, because your brain is constantly at work making new connections, and because you don't know how much basic experience you must pour in before the function begins to click. Also, the breakthrough could come three days after some other session than your first one, and hitting every day creates more third-day opportunities to make the breakthrough. It is much easier to keep track, and to keep to the necessarily rigid and rigorous schedule you set for yourself, if you hit on a daily basis rather than a tri-daily. But don't be surprised if your breakthroughs follow either your initial efforts or your most strenuous efforts by that three-days' interval. Don't miss any scheduled sessions, but make absolutely certain that, three days to the hour following either your initial or a particularly good effort at some "R" or "T" activity, you are at that activity again to take advantage of such possibilities as your brain's three-day gestation period might have opened up.

If you have a medical disability in the area of the function concerned, or run any risk of aggravating a medical problem with that activity, check closely with your physician and work only under his supervision. If such a medical difficulty bars you from a key activity, there is little question but that this can limit the development you can hope to gain from this program, and you will have to work extra hard at other areas to make up for it. But there is plenty of room to work in other areas, and always room for improvement. In the long run there is a solution for the problem of training the brain in the activity which has been barred for medical reasons. That solution involves a special state of Deep Relaxation, the use of that state for *imagining* that forbidden activity, and the use of accelerated subjective time to get in a lot of that imaginary practice. But use of that solution may not be available in your vicinity for some time, so do as does the successful scientist, the successful politician, the successful businessman: go ahead and work with what you already have to work with.

So you are afraid of water or can't bring yourself to get your face in? Then do take lessons, work with a sympathetic instructor, until you can work comfortably in the water. But leave most of your underwater swimming *per se* to the art of learning by fumbling around. Emotionally based fears may also be readily overcome by taking training in any of a number of special disciplines such as Transcendental Meditation, Silva Mind Control, Arica, Scientology, Christian Science, Mind Dynamics, or almost any of a great many others.

Or you can spend money on a psychiatrist, a behavior therapist (an "M-&-M" reward system for getting you to dunk), or a primal scream therapist, or some other clinical and/or exotic psychologist. Or you can procrastinate for years, perhaps, missing all sorts of developmental opportunities until this writer's Psychegenic Learning workshop becomes available in your vicinity. All of which is to say—there are a hundred ways to beat the problem. If you can't get on with it, it's only because you don't really want to.

So now you have scored yourself with an "A," "B," "T," or "R" in medulla mobility, and you have a clear idea of what your developmental needs are on this activity-level and how to provide for them. So also for all the functions to follow: an "A" means you are functioning well and comfortably, a "B" means you find the task uncomfortable but can get along okay, a "T" means you can barely function on this task, and "R" means that you can't handle activities at this level as yet.

When you score an "A," meaning that you are doing fine, further practice in this function and level will still enhance your abilities some, but you have no bottleneck here holding back your development elsewhere.

When you score "B," you need some work on this function and level, on something which has been holding you back in other, perhaps unsuspected regards, but the basic program suggested in this book should suffice.

"T" = Target! Put extra-special effort into developing this function-level and the one just below it. Attacking this bottleneck and opening it up will greatly aid broad areas of the rest of your development.

"R" tells you to regress to the level just below this one and treat that next lower function-level as a "T" area. Every seventy-two hours (three days) during your three-week train-a-thon, make special efforts at the "R" function again to see if you have started to make any progress.

Next to mobility, sight is perhaps the most important activity in your brain. Your infantile medulla, the fish brain that was essentially all that you had working for you when you were born, performs nearly all its visual functions in terms of changes in light value, in terms of changes in light and dark and color.

Rig up a set of flashing Christmas-tree lights, and arrange for these to be the primary source of light in your room while you go on about other things in there. If, while looking at these lights and while doing other things, you feel quite comfortable and indeed find the experience rather pleasant, score yourself an "A" in the Medulla row, second or visual column, on table I.

If you find this experience more or less okay but a bit irritating or distracting after a few minutes, give yourself a "B" in that table. If you experience considerable discomfort, score "T," and for acute discomfort score "R." (Since you have enough use of your eyes to be reading this, it does not seem likely that any reader of this book will score "R" at this point in the table.)

If you experienced discomfort, bring up other lighting in your room relative to the flashing Christmas-tree lights until you reach an arrangement you feel at least somewhat comfortable with, and use this arrangement at frequent intervals. In the event of a "T" score (or an "R"), borrow or acquire a rotating color wheel light such as used in shop-window displays, and use this as your primary source of illumination for a while. More natural devices, such as a breeze-rippled pan of water on your windowsill reflecting sunlight onto your ceiling, or at night looking across a sparkling body of water at lights on the opposite shore, also yield good results.

True, everyday visual experience supplies a considerable number of changes in light value. But it is also true that exercise of higher-brain functions tends to suppress elements of lower-brain functioning. So part of your visual training of your medulla will, sooner or later, depending on your comfort-scoring, consist of looking directly at your flashing Christmas-tree lights for three to five minutes at a time in an otherwise dark room.

Touch actually involves several senses—pressure, heat, cold, pain. Touch is your most immediate sense and is of great importance to your brain's ability to function. If you are reasonably sensitive to even light touches all over your body, score "A." If some areas are rather insensitive or rather hypersensitive, score "B" and give them some extra touch experience during your three-week train-a-thon. Acutely hypersensitive areas, check with your physician. Real numbness anywhere (score "T") rarely fails to react to at least some level of stimulus—sandpaper, blows, pin-pricks, torque, etc.—if the problem is in the brain-mind and not the spinal cord; some stimuli get through, unless there has been definite, traumatic nerve damage.

"T"-level training for touch consists of a barrage of diverse stimuli strong enough to be felt in the numb area. Over time the numb area will become more and more normal.

(No one will score "R"—total body numbness. No brain, and no personality, can develop without at least some sense of touch, and anyone who has traumatically lost all sense of touch will be under such intensive medical care and supervision that anything said here would be superfluous—except that where such numbness is due to stroke or brain disease, many physicians may not yet know that touch [and motor] functions can be restored by a saturation bombardment version of the procedure suggested for "T" just above.)

Motor functions depend upon the sense of touch in large part, as you may have guessed from experiences in which your arm or leg "went to sleep." Other things being equal, the better your sense of touch, the better your condition. Also, the sense of touch appears to involve and activate forms of subliminal pattern-recognition and awareness in the brain such that, other things being equal, the better your sense of touch, the better your personality. And your medulla is functioning at least reasonably well on touch, or you wouldn't be around now to read this book.

Touch is largely suppressed in our society (the reason, perhaps, why most of the world regards us Anglo-Americans as so "cold" and devoid of human personality), though our language, as noted earlier in this book, still recognizes some of touch's supreme importance to our brains. Hearing (despite the roar of traffic and of industrial and household processes) and the functions of speech[1] are not so suppressed. Generally, hearing and speech are not suppressed in our society or in any other major human society. Hearing *is* neurologically deficient in many people, in ways not detected by ordinary hearing tests, which measure hearing sensitivity to sounds of different frequency. Not just hyposensitivity (insensitivity) and hypersensitivity, but what the brain does in interpreting what it hears, are crucial factors. Unless the person overcompensates (usually unconsciously) for hypersensitivity by "tuning out" too much, ordinary hearing tests will not detect hypersensitivity, and in any case will miss the problem area of inadequate brain-handling. The more sophisticated neurologically oriented tests are too involved to repeat here, but you may be able to discover if you have a neurological hearing problem by answering some simple questions. If your answer is yes to several of these questions, neurological hearing may be something of a problem for you and may be worth checking into. If you do discover a problem, you should concentrate a large portion of your three-week train-a-thon on development of hearing. Get your examining physician to tell you which of the four levels of the brain shown on the table is the lowest one associated with the problem, then go to work on *all* functions at that level of the brain, not just the function of hearing. Some of the resulting general development at that level will find its way into the deficient function. Also give some extra work to hearing functions below that level, on the chance that the examining physician, not understanding clearly this neuro-

---

1. Except in the regard that, by discouraging parents or other "amateurs" from teaching early reading to preschoolers, schools are responsible for more than a third of our population today being impaired by reading disabilities. No child taught reading at age one, two or three years of age (some have been successfully started at age six months), by any of a large number of very pleasant and beneficial methods now available for this (see, for example, Glenn Doman's *How to Teach Your Baby to Read,* N.Y.: Random House, 1963), ever has reading problems.

logical approach to the matter, missed something. In any event, extra work below the deficient level will feed some extra development into that level.

Is your answer "yes" to one or more of the following questions?

A. Have you ever been diagnosed, especially in childhood, as having a problem in hearing?

B. When you are tired, does the speech and/or music of other people often tend to fade into gabble?

C. Are noises, talk, music often too soft or uncomfortably loud for you? Is your dynamic range (the range of louds and softs you are comfortable with) narrower than other people's seem to be?

D. Do you, or did you when a child, have more than ordinary difficulty in getting along with other people?

E. When you were a young child, did you and your mother have a less comfortable relationship than others seem to have had? (Too close or too rejecting?)

F. Were you ever clinically diagnosed, as a child, as having emotional or psychological problems?

G. By the standards of those around you, are you pretty much a loner?

H. By the standards of those around you, do you tend to break rules and conventions, appear to others to not really care what others think?

Of course a "yes" answer to any or even all of these questions can arise from many, many different causes besides that of partial, undetected neurologically based hearing deficiencies. But one or more "yes" answers raises the possibility at least and makes the matter worth checking into. Also, many instances of such neurologically based deficiencies, like hyperactivity and autism (two other types of minimal brain-damage dysfunction), cure themselves spontaneously with the passage of time as the brain receives enough input to bridge over the deficiencies. But many don't, or don't completely, cure all traces of the deficiency spontaneously, so "yes" answers to any or several of the above make the matter worth checking into.

You may be wondering about questions D through H. These questions are asked because hearing provides us a lot of awareness besides the communication of speech, and if these awarenesses are missing or impaired, such lacks affect our behavior and personality, especially affecting the way we come across to other people and vice versa. Also, what happens in infancy might be crucial. If, due to a hearing problem, the baby is less than responsive to his mother's voice, she can hardly help but "turn him off" on at least some levels of attitude and relationship. This "turn-off" interferes with the critical "imprinting" phase, in which the baby is first learning to form emotional and interpersonal relationships with other human beings, and forming his model of what it is to be a human being. Anything affecting this critical "imprinting" phase changes the whole spectrum of personality and human relationships. The mother may sense her own "turning off" and overcompensate, creating another spectrum of problems. The mother's (and child's) difficulties are the greatest when the hearing problem is definite but not dramatic enough to be easily detected or even suspected, so that she doesn't know why difficulty exists between her and her child. This problem is the case with most instances of neurological hearing impairment, which is why all young school children and, if possible, preschoolers should be screened for neurological impairments, especially for neurological impairment of hearing, and not just ordinary impairment. Often a child may even be diagnosed as "autistic," and the mother may undeservedly and cruelly castigate herself throughout the rest of her life for having somehow caused the child's "emotional" illness. Therapy for such effects is, of course, beyond the province of this book, and a hundred branches of psychotherapy, analysis, clinical psychology, and exotic disciplines, among other things, are available for rectifying the psychological effects of the problem once correctly identified. (This book does not contain therapy in any form, for that matter, of course, but is an educational description of how to enrich the qualities of your experiencing.)

The difficulties of precise neurological testing of the state of your hearing development, at least at the level on which we are working in this book, are why we have not boxed in the column for hearing. If you answered "yes" to one of the above questions, treat the entire column as "B" and give some added emphasis to the hearing-development aspects of your three-week train-a-thon. If you answered "yes" to "A" or to two or more of the above questions, treat the entire column as "T."

The chemical senses of taste and smell are not critical, but are nice to have. A well-developed sense of smell is probably an assist to having a good memory. If you are, relative to other people, a gourmet, score yourself an "A" throughout the column. If you appear to pretty much lack a sense of taste or smell, score "T" throughout the column. If you appear to completely lack both senses, and nothing—absolutely nothing, not even smelling salts—gets through to you, score "R" and start providing yourself a lot of experience in extremely strong taste (salt, vinegar, honey, lemon) and smell (smelling salts, peppermint or liniment, etc.) stimuli in rapid alternation until things start to get through. If tasty food means little to you, or if you are one of those people who has to have catsup on most meats, score "B" at levels below cortex and "T" in your cortex level for smell and taste. If you can tell odor and taste sensations pretty readily but have trouble identifying them, score yourself "A" for medulla-pons, "B" for midbrain, and "T" for cortex.

Body sense or kinesthesis—a matter of knowing where you are and what you are doing even with your eyes shut and ears stopped—has been given little attention in our society except for athletes (give yourself an "A" all the way up and down the column if you are one) or accident-prone persons, or those who have been diagnosed as having an obvious neurological problem (in either case give yourself a "T" for cortex and midbrain, or an "R" for cortex if the deficiency is a severe one). Because so little attention has been given kinesthetics within the range of everyday experience, it has been more difficult to sort out different levels of kinesthetic experiencing. Nonetheless, you can get some idea of your present functioning and where, if need be, to concentrate your efforts at self-development and bottleneck-removal.

If you can walk successfully, without help, on top of a rail, a fence, or other narrow strip of supporting surface for twenty yards or so and can do so comfortably, give your cortex an "A" for kinesthesia (and for mobility). If you can manage it but find it difficult or uncomfortable, give your cortex a "B." If you can only manage a few feet at a time, give your cortex a "T." If you can't walk without help on that strip even for a few feet, and/or have trouble even standing upon that strip, give your cortex an "R" and your midbrain at best a "T" rating. These are not so much a diagnosis of functioning as they are maps of where and how you will want to work to best effect.

Another test of cortical kinesthesia, and one which makes some distinction between kinesthesis and mobility functions, is to arrange a moderate obstacle course of chairs and tables in your room or elsewhere, and then to make your way around the room without touching anything but with your eyes closed or blindfolded and your ears stopped. That feat rates an "A" for your cortex. Short of "A," the degree of difficulty you experience would determine "B," "T," or "R" rating.

Test your midbrain's kinesthesia by (1) with your eyes closed, bringing your two index fingers together tip-to-tip in that old familiar demonstration, and by (2) making your way around your obstacle course on hands and knees with eyes closed or blindfolded and with ears stopped. Again, a flawless performance scores "A"; the degree of difficulty encountered determines midbrain kinesthetic scores of "B," "T" or "R."

In both cortical and midbrain tests for kinesthesia we have also gotten a measure for mobility. Let us complete our evaluation of your mobility functions as follows:

Cortex. If you get around okay, but if (1) you experience difficulty in running, or if (2) your walking or running gait is awkward or impaired for any reason other than that of definite physical injury, rate your cortex with a "B" instead of an "A" in mobility despite a good kinesthetic performance.

Midbrain. Getting around well and comfortably on all fours—hands and knees—rates "A." Discomfort, awkwardness after several minutes of trial practice to get used to this mode of locomotion, or other difficulties, for reasons other than that of some definite physical injury, rates "B," "T," or "R" depending on how severe the deficiency.

Pons. After a few minutes' practice to get accustomed once again to this primitive mode of locomotion, make your way around stomach-to-floor, keeping as flat as possible. If this gives you difficulty, play an imagination game in which you have suffered a car accident in the middle of a desert, with knee injuries which preclude walking upright or creeping on hands and knees. The oasis of water that will save your life is a hundred yards away. Or you have suffered a combat injury (or are crawling underneath layers of barbed wire entanglement) and a hundred yards of worming your way along the ground will get you back to your own lines and safety. Rest a couple of minutes while you make the imagined situation as real as possible, then start crawling your way toward the oasis or friendly help. If you still experience difficulty in crawling, stomach-to-floor, score your pons with a "B," "T," or "R" according to the extent of that difficulty.

After some practice with pons crawling, if you are getting along well, try doing it around a much smaller obstacle course, eyes shut or blindfolded and ears stopped. If this proves disorienting, rate your pons "B," "T," or "R" on kinesthesia according to the degree of difficulty. Alternatively or in addition, position objects around you on the floor and then, on the floor with eyes shut, slide your arm and hand along the floor and close your hand on the point where you think each object is. Score yourself on the degree of success in this task and do so for both hands, since a deficiency on one side, made difficult to detect at more integrated levels of brain-functioning, can affect other functions almost as broadly as can a detectable deficiency on both sides.

Medulla-level kinesthesia presents interesting problems in assessment, since kinesthesia as experienced anywhere in the levels of brain functioning is barely in the public vocabulary and awareness at all, and because higher-level functions are so difficult to screen out. Perhaps the easiest test for you is that swimming pool again, this time underwater swimming and drifting with eyes shut. Equilibriate your level in the water by means of the amount of air you retain in your lungs, rotate your body a time or so, and then see if you can detect your orientation in the pool, including the directions up and down. If, with practice, you still find yourself somewhat disoriented, rate your medulla's kinesthesia as "B," "T," or "R" and practice this same test activity as a neurologically developing exercise—not only for the sake of neurological development but because of the survival value of being able to orient yourself in water.

(In the event of "R" on this point, the best we can presently suggest is that this activity be practiced while the pool is in sunshine or when there is a great deal of noise in one direction [such as a diving board in action or children playing in the shallow end], or while you are near one of the pool's walls. These methods will give you subliminal orientation while you practice. The associated awarenesses should eventually build up medulla-level kinesthesis where overt, eyes-open impressions would tend to override and screen out kinesthetic awareness at medulla level.)

Are checkerboards or other repetitive outline patterns or motifs particularly uncomfortable to your eyes? Or particularly attractive? In either case give your pons a "B" in the visual column or at worst a "T," since, after all, you are reading, and work accordingly.

Since you are reading, it must be assumed that your cortical vision is in reasonably good shape. If you have difficulties converging your eyes on a common point within three inches or closer, or if you have difficulties tracking rapidly moving objects, or in threading a needle at arm's length (but not at other distances), or if visual complexity is uncomfortable, or if catching a ball is difficult, score your cortex a "B" for vision and work accordingly. If you have trouble tracking movement, or in telling how near or distant objects are, score your midbrain at "B" or "T" and work accordingly.

If reading for any reasonable period of time is difficult or uncomfortable for you, despite reasonably good schooling, don't score any visual function above pons with an "A." (Also, if you wear them, have your glasses checked.) The culprit is usually midbrain functioning, and frequently stems from a person's not having gotten enough hands-and-knees creeping around while he was an infant. Work accordingly.

Can you tell by touch which of the coins in your pocket are nickels, which are dimes, which are pennies? Can you tell by touch which side of the coin is heads and which tails? If the answer to both questions is yes, rate your cortex an "A" on touch. If no to either or both, your cortex gets no better than a "B" in the touch column. It will rate no worse than a "B" if, after putting various small, similar but different objects into a bag, you can tell them apart by touch. If your sense of touch is pretty good at telling things apart, but you have trouble identifying them, as in the exercises of going around in the dark or blindfolded and identifying objects as you come across them, then your midbrain may get an "A" but your cortex a "B" or "T." The table is simplified on this, as on other points, and does not provide for measuring separately the senses of heat, cold, pressure, etc. Nor does it provide for measuring separately your sense of touch in, say, your left foot as distinguished from that in your right hand. If you discover, or have reason to suspect, a deficiency in one of these particular respects, give nothing in the touch columns better than a "B" and work accordingly, and/or check with your nearest available neurologist. Any *new* or recent deficiencies which you realize were not there years before but are now, or older deficiencies which seem to have become greater in recent years, should definitely be checked out with a neurologist and quickly. Chances are excellent that there is no problem, that it was just a matter of letting old functions get rusty, but playing safe is by far the better bet.

Incidentally, as in the peripheral-vision exercises earlier in this book, sophisticating your touch awareness in parts of your body other than your hands represents an easy, accessible, rapidly trainable method of turning on parts of your brain that have been left fallow. To do so (training your left knee to distinguish by touch the skin of a grapefruit from that of an orange, to use a trivial example) will, as in peripheral-vision development, eventually have those additional brain circuits integrating with and participating in the functioning of the main-stream brain functions, in effect giving you more of a brain to work with in those functions.

So now you have filled in the first of the four tables. As you go through the various exercises in this book, write in at the appropriate places on the table any with which you have particular difficulty, and the resulting patterns of notation on the chart will provide you further insights to your brain's functioning and where to concentrate your efforts. For example, if you had difficulty in visually following the figures on the rotating turntable, mark "turntable" on your table for midbrain vision. If in doubt as to where to mark an entry—say, threading a needle at any distance is difficult and you don't know whether to mark this as vision or as kinesthesis—mark it in both. As you go through the exercises in this book, any problems, or any other matters which strike your attention notably, should go into the appropriate place(s) on your chart.

If your self-evaluation gives you nearly all "A's" and no problems, run through your three-week train-a-thon with a fairly even distribution of time through all the exercises. If you encountered problems (you may want to reproduce the self-evaluation table on a larger wall chart to have enough room for your notes), concentrate more of your activity in the affected areas.

Ten days into your three-week train-a-thon, self-evaluate again. Use the second table. You may already see one or two improvements, and this should be encouraging to you. Three days after you have completed your three-week train-a-thon, self-evaluate again—you should see *much* more improvement. The clincher is the fourth table, six weeks after your train-a-thon is concluded. You may have not only retained your gains but, unaware, added new ones as your brain continued to knit

TABLE 1

Self-Evaluation of Brain Functions
Use prior to your three-week train-a-thon

basic level of functions	mobility	vision	touch	hearing	taste/smell	kinesthesis
Cortex						
Midbrain						
Pons						
Medulla						

TABLE 2
Self-Evaluation of Brain Functions
Use midway during your train-a-thon

basic level of functions	mobility	vision	touch	hearing	taste/smell	kinesthesis
Cortex						
Midbrain						
Pons						
Medulla						

TABLE 3
Self-Evaluation of Brain Functions
Use three days after completing your train-a-thon

basic level of functions	mobility	vision	touch	hearing	taste/smell	kinesthesis
Cortex						
Midbrain						
Pons						
Medulla						

TABLE 4

Self-Evaluation of Brain Functions

The clincher—use six weeks after completing your train-a-thon

basic level of functions	mobility	vision	touch	hearing	taste/smell	kinesthesis
Cortex						
Midbrain						
Pons						
Medulla						

its connections from all the new experiences and potentialities you have given it.

Measure your I.Q.? If you want to, go ahead, before, and six to eight weeks after, your train-a-thon. Any psychologist, and almost any school, can either give you an I.Q. test or refer you to someone who will. Or you might save some money and get hold of some of the books that are always kicking around as to how to take examinations—College Boards or S.A.T.s, Civil Service, Graduate Records, etc. Most of these have sample tests you can give yourself, and it is changes in your aptitude scores for which you will be looking. But I.Q. is such a narrow measure of intelligence that the chief value of such testing is simply that of outside, objective confirmation that good things have happened to you since you carried through your three-week train-a-thon. But that confirmation won't be telling you anything. From a far wider, deeper, and richer set of awarenesses and experiencing, you will already *know*.

The world we live in is one of enormous and life-threatening problems. By increasing our own intelligence and that of our fellow man, we increase mankind's ability to solve the pressing problems of the twentieth century.

On a personal level, by increasing your intelligence you provide yourself with a useful tool for helping you to achieve your immediate goals. More important, you leave yourself open to an immense range of life-enhancing possibilities when you increase your awareness of yourself and the world around you.

Suggested Reading

The following are especially recommended for further reading:

Crile, George, Jr. *A Naturalistic View of Man*. New York: World Publishing Company, 1969.

Delacato, Carl. *A New Start for the Child with Reading Problems: A Manual for Parents*. New York: David McKay Co., 1970.

Droscher, Vitus B. *The Magic of the Senses: New Discoveries in Animal Perception*. New York: E. P. Dutton and Co., Inc., 1969.

Ferguson, Marilyn. *The Brain Revolution: The Frontiers of Mind Research*. New York: Taplinger Publishing Company, 1973.

Hunt, J. McVicker. *Intelligence and Experience*. New York: Ronald Press, 1961.

Klosovskii, B. N. *The Development of the Brain, and Its Disturbance by Harmful Factors*. Elmsford, New York: Pergamon, 1963.

Korzybski, Alfred. *Science and Sanity: An Introduction to Non-Aristotelian Systems and General Semantics*. (4th Edition) Lakeville, Connecticut: The International Non-Aristotelian Library Publishing Company, 1958.

Kuhn, Alfred. *The Study of Society: A Unified Approach*. Homewood, Illinois: Irwin-Dorsey, 1963.

Laszlo, Ervin. *A Systems View of the World*. New York: George Braziller Press, 1971.

LeWinn, Edward B. *Human Neurological Organization*. Springfield, Illinois: Charles C Thomas, 1969.

Masters, Robert, and Houston, Jean. *Mind Games: The Guide to Inner Space*. New York: Delta/Dell Publishing Co., 1972.

Pines, Maya. *The Brain Revolution*. New York: Harper and Row, 1973.

Thomas, Evan W. *Brain-Injured Children: With Special Reference to Doman-Delacato Methods of Treatment*. Springfield, Illinois: Charles C Thomas, 1969.

Wenger, Win. *On Raising Human Intelligence*. Federalsburg, Maryland: MCM Press, 1971.

Further useful and relevant information may be found in the following additional bibliography:

Adams, Henry B., Robertson, Malcolm H., and Cooper, David. "Facilitating Therapeutic Personality Changes in Psychiatric Patients by Sensory Deprivation Methods." Private monograph, presented to the International Congress of Psychology, Washington, D.C., 1963.

Altman, J. "Autoradiographic and Histological Studies of Postnatal Neurogenesis. II. A Longitudinal Investigation of the Kinetics and Transformation of Cells Incorporating Tritiated Thymidine in Infant Rats, With Special Reference to Postnatal Neurogenesis in Some Brain Regions." *Journal of Comparative Neurology*. CXXVIII, 1966.

———, and Das, Gopal D. "Autoradiographic Examination of the Effects of Enriched Environment on the Rate of Glial Multiplication in the Adult Rat Brain." *Nature*. CCIV, December 19, 1964. (This was perhaps the earliest significant demonstration that highly developed mammalian adult brains respond in development to increased stimulus almost as dramatically as do infant brains.)

Andrews, A., Belisle, L., Fancy, R., Lortie, R., and Racle, G. "Report of the Canadian Team on Their Stay at the Institute of Suggestology in Sofia." Canadian Public (Civil) Service. Synopsis and translation by staff of Mankind Research Unlimited in Washington, D.C.

Arnold, Arnold. *Teaching Your Child to Learn: From Birth to School Age*. Englewood Cliffs, New Jersey: Prentice-Hall, 1971.

Bagchi, Basu K., and Wenger, Marion A. "Electro-Physiological Correlates of Some Yogi Exercises," *EEG, Clinical Neurophysiology and Epilepsy*. London: Pergamon Press, 1959.

Bailey, Herbert. *Vitamin E: Your Key to a Healthy Heart*. New York: Arc Books, Inc., 1964.

Bancroft, W. Jane. "Foreign Language Teaching in Bulgaria." *Canadian Modern Language Review*. Vol. XXVIII, March, 1972, pp. 8–13.

———. "The Psychology of Suggestopedia, or Learning Without Stress." *The Human Dimensions Institute*. Vol. 2, No. 1, Spring, 1973.

Beck, Joan. *How to Raise a Brighter Child*. New York: Trident, 1967.

Bennett, E. L., Diamond, M. C., Krech, D., and Rosenzweig, M. R. "Chemical and Anatomical Plasticity of the Brain." *Science*. CXLVI, 1964.

———, Krech, D., and Rosenzweig, M. R. "Reliability and Regional Specificity of Cerebral Effects of Environmental Complexity and Training." *Journal of Comparative Physiological Psychology*. LVII, 1964.

Benton, C. D., McCann, J. W., and Larsen, M. "Dyslexia and Dominance." *Journal of Pediatric Opthalmology*. II, 1965.

Benton, W. A., Moser, H., Dodge, P. E., and Carr, S. "Modification of the Schedule of Myelinization in the Rat by Early Nutritional Deprivation." *Pediatrics*. XXXVIII, 1966.

Berelson, Bernard, and Steiner, Gary A. *Human Behavior: An Inventory of Scientific Findings*. New York: Harcourt, Brace and World, Inc., 1964.

Bergamini, L., and Bergamasco, B. *Cortical Evoked Potentials in Man*. Springfield, Illinois: Charles C Thomas, 1967.

Bernstein, Basil. "Social Class and Linguistic Development: A Theory of Social Learning." Halsey, A. H., Floud, Jean, and Anderson, C. A. (eds). *Education, Economy and Society*. New York: The Free Press, 1961.

Bertalanffy, Ludwig von. *General Systems Theory: Foundations, Development, Applications*. New York: George Braziller Press, 1968.

Bertini, M., Lewis, Helen B., and Witkin, Herman A. "Some Preliminary Observations with an Experimental Procedure for the Study of Hypnogogic and Related Phenomena," *Archives of Psychology, Neurology and Psychiatry*. 1964, Vol. 6, 493–534.

Bicknell, F., and Prescott, F. *The Vitamins in Medicine*. New York: Grune and Stratton, 1946.

Bing, Elizabeth. *The Lamaze Method: Six Practical Lessons for an Easier Childbirth*. New York: Grosset and Dunlap, 1957.

Bloom, Benjamin S. *Stability and Change in Human Characteristics*. New York: John Wiley and Sons, 1964.

Boyle, D. G. *A Student's Guide to Piaget*. New York: Pergamon Press, 1969.

Bruner, Jerome S. *The Process of Education*. Cambridge, Massachusetts: Harvard University Press, 1960.

———. *Processes of Cognitive Growth in Infancy*. Heinz Warner Lectures, Clark University, Worcester, Massachusetts, February 8–9, 1963 (private monograph).

———. *Toward a Theory of Instruction*. Cambridge, Massachusetts: Harvard University Press, 1966.

———, Goodenough, Jacqueline J., and Austin, George A. *A Study of Thinking*. New York: John Wiley and Sons, Inc., 1956. Possibly one of the most significant works of our century.

Budzynski, Thomas. "Some Applications of Biofeedback-Produced Twilight States." Paper presented at American Psychological Association Convention, Washington, D.C., 1971.

Cabak, V., and Najdanvic, R. "Effect of Undernutrition in Early Life on Physical and Mental Development." *Archives of Disadvantaged Children*. XL, 1965.

Caulkins, Leroy A. *Normal Labor.* Springfield, Illinois: Charles C Thomas, 1955.

Cazden, Courtney B. "Some Implications of Research in Language Development for Preschool Education." Hess, Robert D., and Bear, Roberta Meyer. *Early Education: Current Theory, Research, and Practice.* Chicago: Aldine Publishing Company, 1968.

Chapman, R. M. "Human Evoked Responses to Meaningful Stimuli." Paper presented to XVIII International Congress of Psychology. Moscow, 1966 (mimeographed paper, privately distributed).

Chase, H. P., Dorsey, J., and McKhann, G. M. "The Effect of Malnutrition on the Synthesis of a Myelin Lipid." *Pediatrics.* XL, 1967.

Cooper, Linn F., and Erickson, Milton H. *Time Distortion in Hypnosis.* Baltimore: Wilkins and Wilkins, 1954.

Cox, Catherine M. "The Early Mental Traits of Three Hundred Geniuses." *Genetic Studies of Genius.* Vol. II. Stanford: Stanford University Press, 1926.

Darlington, F. G., and Chassels, J. B. "Final, Inclusive Report on Five-Year Study on the Effect of Administering Alpha Tocopherol to Thoroughbreds." *Summary.* XII, 1960.

Dart, Raymond A. *Adventures with the Missing Link.* Philadelphia: The Institutes Press, 1967.

Darwin, Charles. *On the Origin of Species by Means of Natural Selection, or The Preservation of Favored Races in the Struggle for Life.* Reprint of 1859 Edition. New York: Philosophical Library, 1951.

Davis, Adelle. *Let's Get Well.* New York: Harcourt, Brace and World, Inc., 1965.

Davison, A. N., and Dobbing, J. "Myelinization as a Vulnerable Period of Brain Development." *British Medical Bulletin.* XXII, 1966.

Deakin, Michael. *The Children on the Hill.* New York: The Bobbs-Merrill Company, Inc., 1972.

Delacato, Carl. *The Diagnosis and Treatment of Speech and Reading Problems.* Springfield, Illinois: Charles C Thomas, 1963.

———. *Neurological Organization and Reading.* Springfield, Illinois: Charles C Thomas, 1966.

———. *The Treatment and Prevention of Reading Problems: The Neuro-Psychological Approach.* Springfield, Illinois: Charles C Thomas, 1959.

Perhaps the first, classic description of Doman-Delacato theory with some of the early procedures, some of which are still important.

———. *The Ultimate Stranger: The Autistic Child.* New York, Doubleday, 1974.

Delgado, Jose M. R. *Physical Control of the Mind: Toward a Psycho-Civilized Society*. New York: Harper and Row, 1969.

Del Giudice, A. "Large Doses of Vitamin E as a Factor in the Mental Improvement of Subnormal Children." *Summary,* XII, 1960.

———. "Massive Doses of Vitamin E as a Factor in Mental Improvement." *Diagnostic Medicine*. XXIX, 1957.

Dennis, W. "Causes of Retardation Among Institutional Children: Iran." *Journal of Genetic Psychology*. XCVI, 1960.

Diamond, M. C., Krech, D., and Rosenzweig, M. R. "The Effects of an Enriched Environment on the Histology of the Rat Cerebral Cortex." *Journal of Comparative Neurology*. CXXIII, 1964.

Dick-Read, Grantly. *Childbirth Without Fear*. New York: Harper and Row, 1944.

Doman, Glenn. *How to Teach Your Baby to Read: The Gentle Revolution*. New York: Random House, 1963.

The classic description of how to teach one- and two-year-olds to read—a tremendously valuable thing to do from the standpoint of brain development, of joyous parent-child relationships, and of preventing future problems in reading (four children in ten who do not learn to read until school age have a life-long reading disability; *none* of the children taught by this or similar methods have any reading problems *if* taught by or before age three years). Infants aged six to eight *months* have been started successfully on reading, and this is an easy method to use.

———. *Treatment Procedures Utilizing Principles of Neurological Organization*. Philadelphia: The Institutes for the Achievement of Human Potential, 1965.

———. *What to Do About Your Brain-Injured Child, or Your Brain-Damaged, Mentally Retarded, Mentally Deficient, Cerebral-Palsied, Emotionally Disturbed, Spastic, Flaccid, Rigid, Epileptic, Autistic, Athetoid, Hyperactive Child*. New York: Doubleday, 1974.

———, and Delacato, Carl. "Doman-Delacato Philosophy." *Human Potential*. I, 1963.

———, Delacato, Carl, and Doman, Robert. *The Doman-Delacato Developmental Language Scale*. Philadelphia: The Rehabilitation Center at Philadelphia, 1961.

———, Delacato, Carl, and Doman, Robert. *The Doman-Delacato Developmental Mobility Scale*. Philadelphia: The Rehabilitation Center at Philadelphia, 1960.

Doman, R. J., Spitz, E., Zucman, E., Delacato, C., and Doman, G. "Children With Severe Brain Injuries." *Journal of the American Medical Association*. CLXXIV, 1960.

Doman, R. J., Taylor, R. G., Jr., and Thomas, E. W. "Brain Injury as a Diagnosis and the Results of Treatment in 335 Brain-Injured Children." *Human Potential.* I, 1968.

Droscher, Vitus B. *The Friendly Beast.* New York: Harper, 1972.

Eccles, J. C. "Possible Ways in Which Synaptic Mechanisms Participate in Learning, Remembering, and Forgetting." *The Anatomy of Memory: Proceedings of the First Annual Conference on Learning, Remembering, and Forgetting.* Palo Alto, California: Science and Behavior Books, 1965.

Ertl, John P. "Evoked Potentials and Intelligence." Lecture delivered by the Director of Cybernetic Studies at University of Ottawa, March 30, 1967, reprinted under the title "Intelligence Testing by Brainwaves." *MENSA Bulletin.* CX, April, 1968.

Evans, Herbert McLean. "Vitamin E." *The Vitamins.* (Anonymously edited.) Evansville, Indiana: Mead, Johnson and Company, undated.

———, and Burr, G. O. "Vitamin E: The Ineffectiveness of Curative Dosage When Mixed With Diets Containing High Proportions of Certain Fats." *Journal of the American Medical Association.* LXXXVIII, 1927.

Eysenck, H. J. "Intelligence Assessment: A Theoretical and Experimental Approach." *The British Journal of Educational Psychology.* XXXVII, February, 1967.

Ferster, C. B., and Perrott, Mary Carol. *Behavior Principles.* New York: Appleton-Century Crofts, 1969.

The first chapter of this book, incidentally, outlines operationally one of the better new teaching techniques to come along, whereby one professor or teacher can give a class of as many as four hundred students much the same kind of intensive and stimulating experience as can normally be done in a small group seminar.

Ferster, C. B., and Skinner, B. F. *Schedules of Reinforcement.* New York: Appleton-Century Crofts, 1957.

Flavell, J. H. *The Developmental Psychology of Jean Piaget.* Princeton: Van Nostrand Co., 1963.

Fredericks, Carlton, and Bailey, Herbert. *Food Facts and Fallacies.* New York: Arc Books, Inc., 1969.

Freud, Sigmund. *A General Introduction to Psychoanalysis.* Garden City, New York: Garden City Publishing Co., 1943.

Galambos, R. "A Glia-neural Theory of Brain Function." *Proceedings of the National Academy of Science.* XLVII, 1961.

Gavalas, R. J., Walter, D. O., Hamer, J., and Adey, W. Ross. "Effect of Low-Level, Low-Frequency Electric Fields in EEG and Behavior in *Macaca* Nemestrina." *Brain Research.* Vol. 18, March 17, 1970, pp. 491–501.

Gesell, A. L., and Amatruda, C. S. *Developmental Diagnosis: Normal and Abnormal Child Development.* New York: Harper, 1947.

Goldfarb, W. "Psychological Privation in Infancy and Subsequent Adjustment." *American Journal of Orthopsychiatry*. XV, 1945.

Gordon, Paul. "Can Inosines Revitalize Our Cells?" *Medical World News*. XI, No. 16, 1970.

Gordon, Thomas. *Parent Effectiveness Training*. New York: P. H. Wyden, 1970.

Gordon, William J. J. *Synectics: The Development of Creative Capacity*. New York: Harper and Row, 1961.

Gray, Susan W., Klaus, Rupert A., Miller, James O., and Forrester, Bettye J. *Before First Grade: The Early Training Project for Disadvantaged Children*. New York: Teachers College Press, 1966.

Guilbaud, G. T. *What Is Cybernetics?* New York: Evergreen Grove Press, 1960.

Guilford, J. P. *The Nature of Human Intelligence*. New York: McGraw-Hill, Inc., 1967.

Guttmacher, Alan F. *Pregnancy and Birth*. New York: Viking, 1956.

Hebb, Donald O. *The Organization of Behavior*. New York: John Wiley and Sons, 1949.

Held, R., and Freedman, S. J. "Plasticity in Human Sensorimotor Control." *Science*. CXLII, 1963.

Held, R., and Hein, A. "Movement-Produced Stimulation in the Development of Visually Guided Behavior." *Journal of Comparative Physiological Psychology*. LVI, 1963.

Held, R., and Rekosh, J. "Motor-Sensory Feedback and the Geometry of Visual Space." *Science*. CXLI, 1963.

Heron, W. T. "The Pathology of Boredom." *Scientific American*. CXCVI, 1957.

Hess, Robert D., and Shipman, Virginia C. "Maternal Influences upon Early Learning: The Cognitive Environments of Urban Pre-School Children." Hess, Robert D., and Bear, Roberta Meyer. *Early Education: Current Theory, Research, and Practice*. Chicago: Aldine Publishing Company, 1968.

Hollingworth, Leta S. *Gifted Children: Their Nature and Nurture*. New York: The Macmillan Company, 1926.

Hooker, D. *Evidence of Prenatal Functions of the Central Nervous System in Man*. James Arthur Lecture on the Evolution of the Human Brain, 1957. New York: The American Museum of Natural History, 1958.

Horney, Karen. *New Ways in Psychoanalysis*. New York: W. W. Norton and Company, 1939.

Horwitt, M. K. "Tocopherol Requirements of Man." *American Journal of Clinical Nutrition*. VIII, 1960.

———, Harvey, C. C., Century, B., and Witting, L. A. "Plasma Tocopherol Hemolysis and Dietary Unsaturated Lipid Relationships in Man." *Federation Proceedings*. XVII, 1958.

Houston, Jean. "Putting the First Man on Earth." *Saturday Review.* No. 204, February 22, 1975, pp. 28–32, 53.

Hubbard, L. Ron. *Dianetics—The Modern Science of Mental Health—A Handbook of Dianetic Procedure.* New York: Saint Hill Press, 1950. Written before commercialization and struggles with the Establishment turned the Dianetics-involved stream of persons and activities into possibly less ideal channels, this book must be regarded with many *caveats,* yet it presents many important techniques that work and that do enhance one's mental capacities to function. Proceed with caution, but proceed.

Hubel, D. H., and Wiesel, T. N. "Single-Cell Responses in Striate Cortex of Kittens Deprived of Vision in One Eye." *Journal of Neurophysiology.* XXVI, 1963.

Human Potential. I, No. 5, 1968.

Hunt, J. McVicker, and Archer, Forough Minou. "An Experimental Study of Psychological Development Before and After Auditory and Visual Enrichments of Orphanage Experience in Young Infants (Draft of Plan for the Program)." Private monograph.

Jensen, Arthur. "Reducing the Hereditary-Environment Uncertainty: A Reply." *Harvard Educational Review.* XXXIX, No. 3, 1969.

Kagan, Jerome. "The Child: His Struggle for Identity." *Saturday Review.* LI, No. 49, December 7, 1968.

Kasamatsu, Akira, and Hirai, Tomio. "An Electroencephalographic Study on the Zen Meditation (Zazen)," *Folio of Psychiatry and Neurology in Japan.* Vol. 20, 1966, pp. 315–336.

Kershner, J. R. "An Investigation of the Doman-Delacato Theory of Neuropsychology as It Applies to Trainable Mentally Retarded Children in Public Schools." Bureau of Research, Administration and Coordination, Area of Research and Development. Department of Public Instruction: Commonwealth of Pennsylvania, 1967.

Krech, David. "In Search of the Engram." *Medical Operations Review.* I, 1966.

———. "Reports of Sections and Societies, General Sessions of the AAAS: Behavior, Brain and Biochemistry." *Science.* CLI, 1966.

———, Crutchfield, Richard S., and Liveon, Norman. *Elements of Psychology.* New York: Alfred A. Knopf, 1969.

———, Rosenzweig, M. R., and Bennett, E. L. "Environmental Improverishment, Social Isolation, and Changes in Brain Chemistry and Anatomy." *Psychology and Behavior.* I, 1966.

———, Rosenzweig, M. R., Bennett, E. L., and Kruekel, B. "Enzyme Concentrations in the Brain and Adjustive Behavior Patterns." *Science.* CXX, 1954.

Kroger, William S. *Childbirth With Hypnosis.* Hollywood, California: Wilshire Book Company, 1968.
One of many methods to have painless childbirth without chemical

anaesthesia. *Any* chemical anaesthesia or analgesia is brain-damaging to the child. The widespread use of such drugs in American obstetrics appears to have cost the average person twenty to thirty points I.Q. Besides hypnosis and self-hypnosis as outlined by Kroger, other methods of painless childbirth include the Birth Suit, Psychegenics, Acupuncture, and (to some extent) LaMaze Natural Childbirth Training. The vertical squatting position is also of some help.

Kubala, A. L., and Katz, M. M. "Nutritional Factors in Psychological Test Behavior." *Journal of Genetic Psychology*. XCVI, 1960.

Langworthy, O. R. "Development of Behavior Patterns and Myelinization of the Nervous System in the Human Fetus and Infant." *Contributions to Embryology*. CXXXIX. Washington: The Carnegie Institution of Washington, Publication No. 443, 1933.

Laski, Marghanita. *Ecstasy: A Study of Some Secular and Religious Experiences*. New York: Cresset (undated).

Laszlo, Ervin. *Introduction to Systems Philosophy: Toward a New Paradigm of Contemporary Thought*. New York: Harper Torchbooks, 1973.

LeBarre, Weston. *The Human Animal*. Chicago: University of Chicago Press, 1964.

Lilly, John C. "Learning Motivated by Subcortical Stimulation: The 'Start' and 'Stop' Patterns of Behavior." Jasper, H. H., Proctor, L. D., Knighton, R. S., Noshay, W. C., and Costello, R. T. *Reticular Formation of the Brain*. Boston: Little, Brown, 1958.

———. *Man and Dolphin*. New York: Pyramid, 1961.

———. "Mental Effects of Reduction of Ordinary Levels of Physical Stimuli on Intact Healthy Persons." *Psychiatric Research Reports*. V, 1956.

Lozanov, Georgi. *Suggestion in Psychology and Education*. New York: Gordon and Breach (publication pending).

Ludwig, Arnold M. "Altered States of Consciousness." *Archives of General Psychiatry*. Vol. 15, 1966, pp. 225–234.

Luria, A. R. *The Working Brain: An Introduction to Neuropsychology* (trans. by Basil Haigh). New York: Basic Books, Inc., 1973.

Maltz, Maxwell. *Psychocybernetics*. Englewood Cliffs, New Jersey: Prentice-Hall, 1960.

Maslow, Abraham H. *Toward a Psychology of Being*. Princeton, New Jersey: Van Nostrand Co., 1962.

Masters, Robert, and Houston, Jean. *Subjective Realities*. Private monograph, 1972.

Mattill, H. A. "The Oxidative Destruction of Vitamin A and E and the Protective Action of Certain Vegetable Oils." *Journal of the American Medical Association*. LXXXIX, 1927.

McCall, R. B. "Stimulus Change in Light-Contingent Bar-Pressing." *Journal of Comparative Physiological Psychology*. LIX, 1965.

McGraw, Myrtle B. *Growth: A Study of Johnny and Jimmy*. New York: Appleton-Century-Crofts, 1935.

Melko, Matthew. *The Nature of Civilizations*. Boston: Porter-Sargent Publisher, 1969.

Melton, David. *The Search for Todd*. Englewood Cliffs, New Jersey: Prentice-Hall, 1968.

Miller, James G. "Living Systems: Basic Concepts." *Behavioral Science*. Vol. 10, No. 3, July 1965, pp. 193–411.

———. "The Nature of Living Systems." *Behavioral Science*. Vol. 16, No. 4, July 1971, pp. 277–301.

———. "Living Systems: The Group." *Behavioral Science*. Vol. 16, No. 4, July 1971, pp. 302–398.

———. "Living Systems: II. The Cell." *Currents in Modern Biology*. No. 4, 1971, pp. 78–206.

———. "Living Systems: III. The Organ." *Currents in Modern Biology*. No. 4, 1971, pp. 207–256.

———. "Living Systems: The Organization." *Behavioral Science*. Vol. 17, No. 1, January 1972, pp. 1–182.

———. "Living Systems: The Organism." *The Quarterly Review of Biology*. No. 3, 1973, pp. 92–276.

Misner, William D. "The Significance of Mobility in Early Childhood: Comparison in Two American Indian Cultures." *Human Potential*. II, No. 1, 1969.

Montessori, Maria. *Spontaneous Activity in Education*. Cambridge, Massachusetts: Robert Bentley, Inc., 1964.

Moore, Omar Khayyam. "On Responsive Environments." Private monograph prepared for the 1967 Abington Conference, "New Directions in Individualizing Instruction." 1967.

———, and Anderson, Alan Ross. *The Responsive Environment: Project*. Pittsburgh: University of Pittsburgh, undated.

———, and Anderson, Alan Ross. "Some Principles for the Design of Clarifying Educational Environments." Goslin, David A. (ed.). *Handbook of Socialization Theory and Research*. New York: Rand McNally and Company, 1969.

Morgan, Clifford T. *Physiological Psychology*. New York: McGraw-Hill, 1965.

Morris, Desmond. *The Naked Ape*. New York: McGraw-Hill, 1967.

Morrow, James. *Mind Meets Matter*. Private monograph, 1970.

Mullahy, Patrick. *Contributions of Harry Stack Sullivan*. New York: Science House, Inc., 1967.

Navarre, John Gabriel. *The Development of Scientific Concepts in a Young Child*. New York: Teachers College Press, 1955.

Newman, Virginia Hunt. *Teaching an Infant to Swim*. New York: Harcourt, Brace and World, 1967.

Ornstein, Robert, and Naranjo, Claudio. *On the Psychology of Meditation.* New York: Viking, 1971.

Osborne, R. T. "Psychometric Correlates of the Visual Evoked Potential." *Acta Psychologica.* XXIX, 1969.

———, Nicora, Barry, and Whitaker, Halford S. *An Analysis of the Human Visual Evoked Response.* Private monograph, undated.

Ostrander, Sheila, and Schroeder, Lynn. *Psychic Discoveries Behind the Iron Curtain.* Englewood Cliffs, New Jersey: Prentice-Hall, Inc., 1970.

Otto, H. A. (ed). *Explorations in Human Potentialities.* Springfield, Illinois: Charles C Thomas, 1966.
A treasure house of new awarenesses.

Pavlov, Ivan P. *Conditioned Reflexes.* London: Oxford University Press, 1927.

Penfield, Wilder. "The Uncommitted Cortex: The Child's Changing Brain." *The Atlantic.* July, 1964.

Perls, Frederick, Hefferline, Ralph F., and Goodman, Paul. *Gestalt Therapy: Excitement and Growth in the Human Personality.* New York: Delta, 1951.

Peters, R. W. "The Effects of Changes in Side-Tone Delay and Level upon the Rate of Oral Reading of Normal Speakers." *Journal of Speech and Hearing Disorders.* XIX, 1954.

Piaget, Jean. *The Origins of Intelligence in Children.* New York: W. W. Norton and Co., 1963.
This was the classic study that today is revolutionizing wide sectors of psychology and education.

Pines, Maya. *Revolution in Learning.* New York: Harper and Row, 1966.

Pribram, Karl H. *Languages of the Brain.* Englewood Cliffs, New Jersey: Prentice-Hall, 1971.

Prudden, Bonnie. *Your Baby Can Swim.* Reader's Digest Press (Distributed by E. P. Dutton, Co., Inc., New York, 1974.)

Rapoport, Anatol. *Science and the Goals of Man.* New York: Harper and Brothers, 1943.

Riesen, A. H. "Studying Perceptual Development Using the Technique of Sensory Deprivation." *Journal of Nervous Mental Disorders.* CXXXII, 1961.

Rimland, Bernard. "*Infantile Autism: The Syndrome and Its Implications for a Neural Theory of Behavior.* New York: Appleton-Century Crofts, 1964.

Rodale, J. I. *Natural Health and Pregnancy: A Handbook for Mothers-to-Be.* New York: Pyramid Books, 1968.

Rogers, Carl R. *On Becoming a Person.* Boston: Houghton Mifflin Company, Sentry Edition, 1961.

Rosenzweig, M. R., Krech, D., Bennett, E. L., and Diamond, M. C.

"Effects of Environmental Complexity and Training on Brain Chemistry and Anatomy: A Replication and Extension." *Journal of Comparative Physiological Psychology*. LV, 1962.

Rubin, F. "*Learning and Sleep: The Theory and Practice of Hypnopaedia*." New York: John Wright, 1971. For all the popular interest in sleep-learning, there is precious little useful literature available on it, as evidenced by weaknesses in this, presumably a leading text on the subject.

Russell, Bertrand. *The Problems of Philosophy*. (From 1912.) New York: Oxford University reprint, 1972.

Scheibel, M. E., and Scheibel, A. B. "Some Structural-Functional Correlates of Development in Young Cats." *EEG Clinical Neurophysiology* XXIV (Supplement), 1963.

Scott, J. P., Fredericson, E., and Fuller, J. L. "Experimental Exploration of the Critical Period Hypothesis." *Personality*. I, 1951.

Selye, Hans. *The Stress of Life*. New York: McGraw-Hill, 1956.

Sharp, Evelyn. *Thinking Is Child's Play*. New York: E. P. Dutton and Company, 1969.

Shute, Evan. "The Current Status of Alpha Tocopherol in Cardiovascular Disease." Bailey, Herbert. *Vitamin E: Your Key to a Healthy Heart*. New York: Arc Books, Inc., 1965.

———. *The Heart and Vitamin E*. London, Ontario: Evan Shute Foundation for Medical Research, 1969.

Singh, Jagjit. *Information Theory, Language and Cybernetics*. New York: Dover, 1966.

Spitz, René A. "Hospitalism: An Inquiry into the Genesis of Psychiatric Conditions in Early Childhood." Eissler, R. S., Freud, A., Hartmann, H., and Kris, E. (eds.). *The Psychoanalytic Study of the Child*. New York: International University Press, 1945, Vol. I.

Stone, L. Joseph, and Church, Joseph. *Childhood and Adolescence: A Psychology of the Growing Person*. New York: Random House, 1957.

Strean, Lyon P. *The Birth of Normal Babies*. New York: Twayne, 1958.

A Summary of Concepts, Procedures and Organization. Philadelphia: The Institutes for the Achievement of Human Potential, 1964.

Sutherland, Robert L., Woodward, Julian L., and Maxwell, Milton A. *Introductory Sociology*. Philadelphia: Lippincott, 1961.

Suzuki, Shinichi. *Nurtured by Love*. New York: Exposition Press, 1969.

——— (ed.). *The Suzuki Symposium on Early-Childhood Education*. New York: Music School of the Henry Street Settlement, 1967.

Szasz, Anna. "Vitamin E in the Treatment of Mongolian Idiocy. Influence on the Organism of Vitamin E Given from Birth Onward Until Puberty." *Summary*. XI, 1959.

Tanner, J. M., and Inhelder, B. (eds.). *Discussions on Child Development.* New York: International University Press, 1953, Vol. I.

Tart, Charles T. (ed.). *Altered States of Consciousness.* Garden City, N.Y.: Doubleday-Anchor, 1972. Tart's own theory is weak, but much of the content of this book is illuminating.

Tasaki, I., and Chang, J. J. "Electric Responses of Glia Cells in Cat's Brain." *Science.* CXXVIII, 1958.

Terman, Lewis M. *Genetic Studies of Genius.* Stanford: Stanford University Press. 1926.

Teyler, Timothy J. (ed.). *Altered States of Awareness: Readings from Scientific American.* 1972.

Thomas, Roger K., Jr. *Problems and Procedures in Correlating Electrical Brain Activity with Cognition.* Louisville, Kentucky: Southern Society for Philosophy and Psychology, 1968.

Thompson, W. R., and Heron, W. "The Effects of Restricting Early Experience on the Problem-Solving Capacity of Dogs." *Canadian Journal of Psychology.* VIII, 1954.

Van Bergeijk, W. A., and David, E. E. "Delayed Handwriting." *Perceptual Motor Skills,* IX, 1959.

Vogel, W., Broverman, D. M., Klaiber, E. L., Kobayashi, Y., Abraham, G., and Broverman, Inge K. *EEG, Androgens, and Mental Abilities.* Louisville, Kentucky: Southern Society for Philosophy and Psychology, 1968.

Vygotsky, Lev. *Thought and Language.* Cambridge, Massachusetts: The M.I.T. Press, 1962.

Wallace, Robert Keith. *The Physiological Effects of Transcendental Meditation.* Dissertation thesis, UCLA, 1970.

Ward, Virgil S. *Educating the Gifted: An Axiomatic Approach.* Columbus, Ohio: Charles E. Merrill Books, Inc., 1961.

Wei, King D. "Comparative Effects of Certain Antioxidants on Gestational Performance and Teratogeny in Vitamin-E-Deficient Rats." *Journal of Nutrition.* LXXXII, 1964.

Wenger, Win. "Distinctiveness Amidst a Calm." *PIC'NS.* I, 1970.

———. "Infant Reading: Sesame Street and Glenn Doman." *MENSA Research.* I:5, December 1970.

———. "May People Become Significantly Abler to Share More Fully the Human Experience? Report of a MENSA Symposium on Raising Human Intelligence." *MENSA Research.* I:4, June 1970.

———. "On the Pathology of Civilizations." *MENSA Research* I:6, 1971.

———, and members of the staff of Mankind Research Foundation. *Program to Test Cue-Reinforced Learning (CRL) Technique.* Private monograph. 1973.

———, and members of the staff of Mankind Research Foundation.

Test of Two Learning Methods. Proposal and private monograph. 1974.

———. *The TRAHI Report: Report of the Team for Research in Augmenting Human Intelligence.* 5 issues. Federalsburg, Maryland: MCM Press, 1971.

———. "Intelligence and Vitamin E." *MENSA Bulletin* No. 148, September 1971.

———. "Returns from Parents Support Vitamin E Proposition: A Reply to Theodore Cogswell's Letter." *MENSA Bulletin* No. 154, March 1972.

———. *The Organic Analogy in Human Society: A Re-Examination.* Private monograph. Rockville, Maryland: MCM Press, 1973. Originally prepared for an address of the "Civilizations as Systems" session of the December 1972 Washington, D.C., Conference of the American Association for the Advancement of Science. Contains a very succinct summary of General Systems Theory.

White, Burton L. "An Experimental Approach to the Effects of Experience on Early Human Behavior." Hill, J. P. (ed.). *Minnesota Symposium on Child Psychology.* Minneapolis: University of Minnesota Press, 1967.

———. "The Initial Coordination of Sensori-Motor Schema in Human Infants—Piaget's Ideas and the Role of Experience." Elkind, D., Davis, A., and Flavell, John (eds.). *Studies in Cognitive Development: Essays in Honor of Jean Piaget.* New York: Oxford University Press, 1967.

———, and Held, R. "Plasticity of Sensori-Motor Development in the Human Infant." Rosenblith, J. F., and Allinsmith, W. (eds.). *The Causes of Behavior: Readings in Child Development and Educational Psychology.* Boston: Allyn and Bacon, 1966.

Weiner, Norbert. *Cybernetics and Society: The Human Use of Human Beings.* New York: Doubleday Anchor Books, 1954.

Williams, Roger J. *Biochemical Individuality.* New York: John Wiley and Sons, 1956.

———. *Nutrition Against Disease.* New York: Bantam Books, Inc., 1973.

Young, J. Z. *A Model of the Brain.* London: Oxford University Press, 1964.